DIABETES MEALS
ON $7 A DAY–OR LESS!
2ND EDITION

How to Plan Healthy Menus without Breaking the Bank

Patti B. Geil, RD, CDE, MS, FADA, and
Tami A. Ross, RD, LD, CDE

American Diabetes Association®
Cure • Care • Commitment®

Director, Book Publishing, Rob Anthony; *Managing Editor*, Abe Ogden; *Editor*, Rebekah Renshaw; *Production Manager,* Melissa Sprott; *Composition*, ADA; *Cover Design*, VC Graphics; *Printer:* Thomson–Shore, Inc.

Printed in the United States of America
1 3 5 7 9 10 8 6 4 2

The suggestions and information contained in this publication are generally consistent with the *Clinical Practice Recommendations* and other policies of the American Diabetes Association, but they do not represent the policy or position of the Association or any of its boards or committees. Reasonable steps have been taken to ensure the accuracy of the information presented. However, the American Diabetes Association cannot ensure the safety or efficacy of any product or service described in this publication. Individuals are advised to consult a physician or other appropriate health care professional before undertaking any diet or exercise program or taking any medication referred to in this publication. Professionals must use and apply their own professional judgment, experience, and training and should not rely solely on the information contained in this publication before prescribing any diet, exercise, or medication. The American Diabetes Association—its officers, directors, employees, volunteers, and members—assumes no responsibility or liability for personal or other injury, loss, or damage that may result from the suggestions or information in this publication.

⊗ The paper in this publication meets the requirements of the ANSI Standard Z39.48-1992 (permanence of paper).

ADA titles may be purchased for business or promotional use or for special sales. To purchase more than 50 copies of this book at a discount, or for custom editions of this book with your logo, contact Lee Romano Sequeira, Special Sales & Promotions, at the address below, or at LRomano@diabetes.org or 703-299-2046.

For all other inquiries, please call 1-800-DIABETES.

American Diabetes Association
1701 North Beauregard Street
Alexandria, Virginia 22311

Library of Congress Cataloging-in-Publication Data
Geil, Patti Bazel.
  Diabetes meals on $7 a day—or less / Patti Geil and Tami Ross.—2nd ed.
    p. cm.
  Includes bibliographical references and index.
  ISBN-13: 978-1-58040-272-9 (alk. paper) 41935221   10/09
  1. Diabetes--Diet therapy--Recipes. 2. Low budget cookery. I. Ross, Tami. II. Title.
III. Title: Diabetes meals on seven dollars a day-- or less.
  RC662.G45 2007
  641.5'6314--dc22

                    2007015972

CONTENTS

ACKNOWLEDGMENTS

To Jack, Kristen, and Rachel: Your love and support is priceless!

—Patti B. Geil

To my Mother, who instilled in me at an early age the value of a dollar. Thank you for teaching me always to spend my money wisely.

—Tami A. Ross

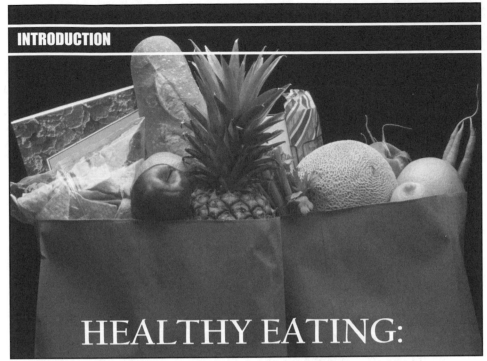

HEALTHY EATING:
A Blue-Chip Investment

I t is just a quick trip to the supermarket to pick up a few things. You reach the checkout line and you're suddenly slammed with sticker shock. How could just a few bags of groceries cost more than $100? You know that healthy eating is vital for people with diabetes, yet once again you find yourself thinking, "I can't afford to eat healthfully."

Without a doubt, diabetes is an expensive disease. One out of every 10 health care dollars spent in the United States is spent on diabetes and its complications. Family budgets must stretch to cover the costs of medications, monitoring supplies, and more frequent visits to health care providers. People with diabetes spend $13,243 annually on health care, compared to those without diabetes who spend only $2,560 each year.

It is a common misconception that a healthy diabetes diet must be costly and consist of special diabetic foods and high-priced sugar-free treats. American households already spend 14 cents of every dollar of their disposable income on food. Given the additional expenses associated with proper medical management of diabetes, revising your meal planning and shopping strategies will save you money without shortchanging your health.

Investing a bit of time and money in healthy eating is a blue-chip invest-ment for your future. Results of the Diabetes Control and Complications Trial (DCCT) showed that improving blood glucose control lowers the risk of diabetes complications—such as eye and kidney disease—in individuals with type 1 diabetes. The United Kingdom Prospective Diabetes Study (UKPDS) showed similar results in patients with type 2 diabetes.

Nutrition is a key factor in helping to control your diabetes. Spending the money to eat healthfully will improve blood glucose control now and may help prevent costly complications and expensive medical care later in life.

Eating well and spending less are not mutually exclusive. In fact, healthi-er foods can actually save you money. Researchers have found that when families went on weight loss diets, they not only lost weight but also reduced their food budgets. The savings came from reducing portion sizes and buying fewer high-calorie, high-priced foods. If you think you must buy expensive special versions of the foods your family usually eats, think again! The American Diabetes Association nutrition recommendations sim-ply suggest eating healthfully—the same advice that already applies to every member of your family.

The nutrition guidance for people with diabetes is the same as that for anyone interested in eating healthfully. It consists of a plate full of low-fat, high-fiber grains, beans, fruits, and vegetables with small portions of meat and protein foods and limited amounts of fats, sweets, and alcohol. Everyone should strive to eat according to these guidelines to lower the risk of heart disease, obesity, and some forms of cancer. Involve your fam-ily in your healthy eating, cost-cutting campaign. Your family—and your wallet—will thank you for it.

So leave those costly diet or diabetic foods on the grocery store shelf. Hands off the high-priced sugar-free sweets. The latest nutrition recom-mendations give you the freedom to enjoy small amounts of regular sugar and sweets, as long as your weight, blood glucose levels, and blood lipids remain in control. If you are used to spending significant amounts of money on artificially sweetened treats, you can use your savings to invest in another treat—like a new exercise video or a stress-free evening out on the town.

SPEND LESS, EAT HEALTHFULLY

Now, more than ever, eating healthfully on a budget is a challenge. When we first published *Diabetes Meals on $7 a Day—or Less!* in 1999, the American Farm Bureau Federation Marketbasket Survey showed that purchasing 16 basic grocery items costs $32.51. Today, those same 16 items ring up at $42.95. The good news is that you can eat a wide variety of healthy foods without breaking the bank. The American Dietetic Association has demonstrated that a 2,000-calorie meal plan costs approximately $6.69 per person per day and only $6.33 if you're a vegetarian. You will find that the more time and effort you're willing to spend, the more money you're likely to save. For example, it may take a few extra moments to prepare quick cooking oats rather than the microwave instant version, but the trade off of time for money and good health is worth it.

ATTENTION SHOPPERS! ECONOMICAL EATING IN AISLE ONE

The American Dietetic Association has calculated the average daily costs to eat according to the 2005 Dietary Guidelines for Americans.

Recommendation: 4 1/2 cups of fruits and vegetables
(Fresh strawberries, bananas, spinach, romaine lettuce, carrots; frozen blueberries, broccoli, cauliflower; canned peaches) **$2.12**

Recommendation: 6 ounces of grains
(Oatmeal, brown rice, whole-wheat bread) **$0.88**

Recommendation: 3 cups of fat-free or low-fat milk or equivalent
(Yogurt, fat-free milk, cheese) **$1.60**

Recommendation: 5 1/2 ounces of protein
(Cooked lean beef, chicken, pork, or ground turkey; eggs; fresh fish) **$1.72**

Recommendation: 6 teaspoons of fats
(Olive oil, vegetable oil, light salad dressing, low-fat mayonnaise) **$0.37**

TOTAL = $6.69 per day

Economical diabetes meal planning doesn't mean deboning countless chickens, serving endless meals of leftovers, or driving all over town for grocery store specials. You can even take an occasional night off kitchen duty for a carefully chosen fast-food meal. But keep in mind that drive-through deals may have hidden costs.

While upsizing a meal costs you only $0.67 for 400 extra calories from fries and soda, it may be draining your wallet in unexpected ways. For every 100 calories a person eats beyond his or her daily needs, the price of food, medical care, and gasoline—heavier passengers reduce a car's fuel efficiency—rises anywhere from $0.48 to nearly $2. The heavier a person is, the greater the cost. Fast-food deals may not be deals at all. The tips in Chapter 6 will enable you to enjoy eating out while still watching your nutritional and financial budgets.

Everyone loves to save money, no matter what his or her bank account balance. *Diabetes Meals on $7 a Day—or Less!, 2nd Edition* will guide you in your quest to eat healthfully on a lean budget. The recipes are quick and simple to assemble, and contain easy-to-find ingredients.

If you are eligible for food assistance programs, such as food stamps, WIC (Women, Infants, and Children), or Meals-on-Wheels, you'll find that the recipes and menus in this book will help you make the most of the foods available through these sources. Pick a few new recipes, take a look at the meal plans, and review the shopping tips before your next trip to the supermarket. You may be pleasantly surprised to find that the small changes we suggest will quickly add up to make you healthier and wealthier.

Money $aving Tip

Saving just $5 a week on food can fatten your piggy bank by more than $250 a year. You can spend less and eat healthy!

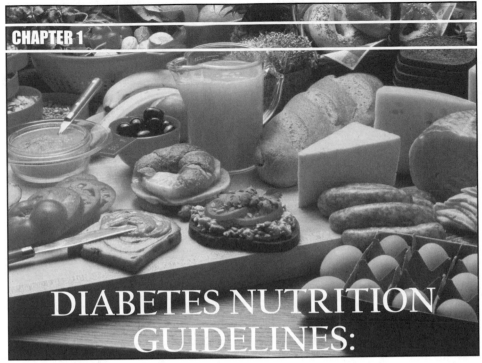

CHAPTER 1

DIABETES NUTRITION GUIDELINES:

HEALTHY, WEALTHY, AND WISE

Do you think the right foods for your diabetes are too costly for your family's food budget? Maybe you mistakenly believe some of these common diabetes money myths:

- "I can't afford to follow a diabetes meal plan. It's too expensive."
- "I'll have to spend too much on special foods that the rest of my family won't eat."
- "I can't pay for all the fresh fruits and vegetables and high-priced cuts of meat a diabetes meal plan requires."

This book was created to dispel these myths and prove that good food does not have to break your budget. Eating foods that are healthy for diabetes should cost you only a bit more than you're already spending in time, effort, and dollars.

Good Food for the Entire Family

If you are concerned that your diabetes nutrition needs will stretch the family's food budget, don't worry. The latest diabetes nutrition recommendations parallel the most recent dietary guidelines, which emphasize making smart choices from every food group, finding a balance between food and physical activity, and getting the most nutrition out of your calories.

Adequate Nutrients Within Calorie Needs

Consuming a variety of nutrient-dense foods and beverages within the basic food groups is the best way to ensure you will meet all of your nutrient needs. It is also important to limit your intake of saturated and trans fats, cholesterol, added sugars, salt, and alcohol.

Weight Management

In order to maintain your weight in a healthy range, balance calories from foods and beverages with calories expended. To prevent gradual weight gain over time, make small decreases in food calories and increase physical activity.

Physical Activity

Engaging in regular physical activity and reducing sedentary activities promotes health, psychological well-being, and a healthy body weight. The best way to achieve physical fitness is by incorporating cardiovascular conditioning, with stretching exercises for flexibility, and resistance exercises or calisthenics for muscle strength and endurance into your workout.

- To reduce the risk of chronic disease in adulthood, engage in at least 30 minutes of moderate-intensity physical activity on most days of the week. Greater health benefits can be obtained by engaging in physical activity of more vigorous intensity or longer duration.
- To help manage body weight and prevent weight gain, engage in 60 minutes of moderate- to vigorous-intensity activity on most days of the week while not exceeding caloric intake requirements.
- To sustain weight loss in adulthood, participate in at least 60–90 minutes of daily moderate-intensity physical activity, while not exceeding caloric intake requirements. You may need to consult a health care provider before participating in this level of activity.

Food Groups to Encourage

Fats

■ Consume less than 7% of calories from saturated fatty acids and less than 200 mg/day of cholesterol. Try to keep trans fatty acid consumption as low as possible.

■ Keep total fat intake between 20 and 35% of calories, with most fats coming from sources of polyunsaturated and monounsaturated fatty acids—such as fish, nuts, and vegetable oils.

■ When selecting and preparing meat, poultry, dry beans, and milk or milk products, make choices that are lean, low fat, or fat free.

■ Limit intake of foods that contain fats and oils high in saturated and/or trans fatty acids.

Carbohydrates

■ Include fiber-rich fruits, vegetables, and whole grains as part of your everyday diet.

■ Choose and prepare foods and beverages with little added sugars or caloric sweeteners. Use the U.S. Department of Agriculture (USDA) Food Guide and the DASH Eating Plan for reference.

■ Reduce the incidence of dental caries by practicing good oral hygiene and consuming less sugar and starch containing foods and beverages.

Sodium and potassium

- Consume less than 2,300 mg—approximately 1 tsp—of sodium per day.
- Choose and prepare foods with little salt. At the same time, consume potassium-rich foods like fruits and vegetables.

Alcoholic beverages

Those who choose to drink alcoholic beverages should do so sensibly and in moderation—defined as the consumption of one drink per day for women and up to two drinks per day for men. Make sure to check your blood glucose after consumming alcohol because alcohol can raise certain blood fats and may cause low blood glucose.

ALCOHOL AWARENESS

Alcoholic beverages should never be consumed by certain individuals, including:

- those who cannot restrict their alcohol intake
- women of childbearing age who may become pregnant
- pregnant and lactating women
- children and adolescents
- individuals taking medications that can interact with alcohol
- those with specific medical conditions
- individuals engaging in activities that require attention, skill, or coordination, such as driving or operating machinery

Food Safety

To avoid microbial foodborne illness:

- Clean hands, food contact surfaces, and fruits and vegetables.
- Separate raw, cooked, and ready-to-eat foods while shopping, preparing, or storing foods.
- Cook foods to a safe temperature to kill microorganisms.
- Chill (refrigerate) perishable food promptly and defrost foods properly.
- Avoid raw (unpasteurized) milk and any products that may contain unpasteurized milk. Foods containing raw eggs, undercooked meat, unpasteurized juices, and raw sprouts should also be avoided.

DIABETES FOOD GOALS FOR YOU

The first diabetes diet recommendations were made in Egypt in 1550 B.C., and consisted of wheat grains, fresh grits, grapes, honey, and sweet beer. Today, the American Diabetes Association nutrition recommendations stress an overall healthy eating plan, with an emphasis on several vital nutrients.

If you'd like to learn more about specific nutrient needs and food recommendations for your family members based on gender, age, and activity level, access the website of the USDA's new interactive food model, MyPyramid, at *www.mypyramid.gov.*

Calories

The days of preprinted, calorie-level diet sheets are over. Although we know that most adults require between 1,800 and 2,500 calories per day, what you need to maintain a reasonable body weight may be different. To lose weight, between 1,000 and 1,600 calories per day may be your goal. Individualized meal plans, designed with the help of a registered dietitian (RD), are the best for watching your weight.

Protein

Your intake of protein foods (meats, poultry, seafood, dairy foods, beans, peas, nuts, and seeds) should be at the same level as that of the general public. These foods should make up between 15 and 20% of the calories you eat, which translates into two 3-oz servings each day (3 oz is the size of a deck of cards or the palm of a woman's hand).

Although a high intake of protein may be a risk factor for the development of diabetic kidney disease, there is evidence that vegetable protein—which comes from beans, grains, and vegetables—may slow the rate of kidney disease in people with diabetes. Eating less protein from animal sources—meat, milk, eggs, and cheese—also means less fat, saturated fat, and cholesterol in your diet.

Fat

A lower fat intake also lowers your risk for cardiovascular (heart) disease, a common complication of diabetes. Lower fat intake means lower calorie intake, which helps you maintain a reasonable body weight. Mono- and polyunsaturated fats can help to lower your blood cholesterol and protect your heart. Saturated and trans fats can raise your blood cholesterol and increase your risk of heart disease.

The cholesterol in food may also increase your blood cholesterol. Limiting your intake of animal proteins and whole-milk dairy foods will help you to consume less fat and cholesterol in your diet. Your cholesterol intake should be less than 200 milligrams per day. Intake of trans fat and saturated fat should be minimized. The exact amount and type of fat you should eat will depend on your weight, your blood lipid levels, and your overall health.

Carbohydrates

Carbohydrates from fruits, vegetables, whole grains, legumes, and low-fat milk are great for your health. Sweets can be substituted for other carbohydrates in your meal plan or covered with insulin or other glucose-lowering medications.

Both the amount (grams) of carbohydrates as well as the type of carbohydrates in a food influence your blood glucose levels. Monitoring your total grams of carbohydrates—whether by using the exchanges/choices system or carbohydrate counting—is a great strategy to help improve your blood glucose control.

There is no need for you to spend money on special diabetic foods unless you enjoy their taste or the variety they provide. Sweeteners such as corn syrup, fruit juice, and sorbitol may offer no advantage over regular sugar. Enjoy sweet treats in moderation. Substitute sweets for other carbohydrates in your diet, and check your blood glucose after eating to see how they affect you.

Fiber

You should be eating the same amount of fiber as the other members of your family—approximately 20–35 grams per day, or 14 g for every 1,000 calories you eat. Unfortunately, most Americans eat only 10–13 grams daily, so they don't reap all of fiber's benefits, like better digestive health. To ensure you are getting the most out of fiber in your diet, choose whole-wheat grains and plenty of fresh fruits and vegetables every day. Oats and dried beans are great sources of soluble fiber, which has a positive effect on blood lipid levels.

Sodium

Sodium intake recommendations for people with diabetes are similar to those for the general population—less than 2,300 milligrams per day. If you have high blood pressure, it may be helpful to eat less, shake the salt habit, and carefully read food labels to track the amount of sodium in your diet.

Sweeteners

FDA-approved reduced-calorie sweeteners include sugar alcohols, such as sorbitol, xylitol, and hydrogenated starch hydrolysates. Keep in mind that reduced-calorie sweeteners contain both calories and carbohydrates.

The FDA has approved five nonnutritive (zero calorie) sweeteners for use in the U.S. They are:

- acesulfame potassium
- aspartame
- neotame
- saccharin
- sucralose

Vitamins and Minerals

You may be a good candidate for vitamin and mineral supplements if you are in poor diabetes control; if you are on a very restricted weight-loss diet; if you are elderly, pregnant, or breast-feeding; or if you are a strict vegetarian.

Eating a well-balanced diet should provide everyone with the essential vitamins and minerals they require. At this time the American Diabetes Association does not recommend any special supplements to benefit individuals with diabetes, however, you should ask your health care team to discuss your individualized vitamin and mineral needs.

Smart Choices

The ever-changing information about diabetes nutrition may have left you more confused than ever. A session with an RD and certified diabetes educator (CDE) is money and time well invested. An RD can evaluate your individual case and suggest the meal planning approach that is best for you, whether it is the MyPyramid, carbohydrate counting, or something in between.

Making smart food choices is the key to taking care of your diabetes. Poor choices will cost you time, money, and your health. Eating well helps you avoid the expensive damage to your eyes, heart, and kidneys that occurs when blood glucose levels are high day after day. You can eat healthfully on a lean budget by using the diabetes nutrition guidelines to make smart food choices.

ADDITIONAL RESOURCES IN YOUR AREA

- To find an RD near you, call The American Dietetic Association at 1-800-877-1600 or visit the website *www.eatright.org*. Ask for a specialist in diabetes nutrition.
- To find a CDE in your area, call the American Association of Diabetes Educators at 1-800-338-3633 or visit the website *www.aadenet.org*.
- To find a diabetes education program in your area, call 1-800-342-2383 or log onto the American Diabetes Association's website at *www.diabetes.org*.

MOTHER NATURE KNOWS BEST

Sticking to the most basic, natural, and nutritious foods is far better for both your health and pocketbook than ready-to-eat, highly processed, and expensive refined foods.

Refined, Processed Food	Better Choice
soda, soft drinks, fruit drinks	Water, unsweetened fruit juice, low-fat milk
sweetened cereal	whole-grain and unsweetened cereal
candy	homemade trail mix (dried fruit, nuts, and sunflower seeds)
snack chips	popcorn, dry roasted nuts
salad dressing	homemade oil, vinegar, and herbs; low-fat mayonnaise; or plain yogurt

Keep this example in mind: Five pounds of naturally fat-free baking potatoes costs $2.79. In contrast, you'll pay $16.50 for 5 pounds of high-fat potato chips. It's easy to see which choice is better for your budget—and your health!

Money $aving Tip

Regular physical activity works to promote good health, helping to lower the cost of medical bills in the future.

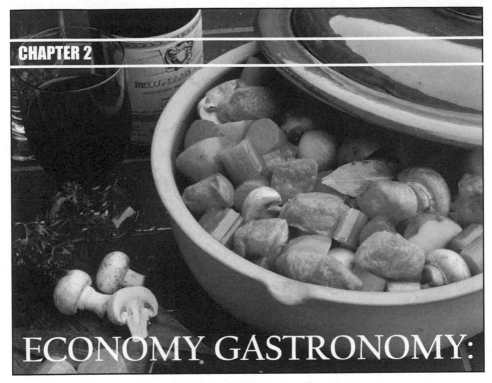

CHAPTER 2

ECONOMY GASTRONOMY:

Penny-Wise Meal Planning, Cost-Wise Cooking

P enny-wise meal planning and cost-wise cooking are the first steps
to stretching your food dollar while eating healthfully. The USDA
has estimated that a family of four can eat at home for a cost of
just $102.40 to $119.10 a week. That's only $3.66 to $4.25 per person per
day—the price of just one fast food value meal. Sound impossible? It's
not. For more information on economical eating, check out the USDA
website at *www.usda.gov*, for sample food plans to match your individualized
budget requirements.

   Eating healthfully on a lean budget does require a small investment of
time to plan meals for the week and cook the foods that match your budget and diabetes nutrition requirements. But, the little amount of extra time
you spend is an investment that can really make a difference when trying to
cut costs.

PENNY-WISE MEAL PLANNING

Like most people, you are probably pressed for time and often eat meals on the run. Why should you use even a few of your precious moments for meal planning? When you consider that food costs are usually the second largest monthly expense—after mortgage or rent payments—reducing that expense can raise the budget savings significantly. Take a closer look at the long-term savings in money, time, and health that come with taking the time to think ahead about what you'll be eating.

SEVEN SIMPLE STEPS TO MEAL PLANNING

1. Determine your food budget.
2. Decide how often you will shop.
3. Know how many people will be eating each meal so you don't buy too much food.
4. Plan breakfast, lunch, dinner, and snacks incorporating store specials. Stay flexible so that you can switch meals around if your plans change at the last minute.
5. Check what's in the pantry, then make a list of ingredients that you need to purchase to prepare each meal and snack.
6. Keep the shopping list handy in the kitchen and add to it during the week as you run out of staples.
7. Make meal planning a habit.

How Planning Meals Helps

Planning your meals a week in advance enables you to:

- **Provide healthy meals for you and your family.** When meals are planned ahead, you can be sure that the meals are balanced.
- **Take advantage of special sales.** Review your newspaper's grocery store advertisements and find foods that fit your budget. Plan meals around the specials for the week to take a bite out of your expenses.
- **Grocery shop from a list.** Studies show that without a list in hand you can spend almost twice as much at the store.
- **Resist impulse buying.** If you know what you need for the week and stick to your list, you are more likely to avoid high priced/low nutrition items like snack chips and sugar-free candy.

- **Save time.** By planning meals in advance you'll be able to do all of your shopping at one time. You won't have to make several trips to the store to buy foods you forgot, which translates into gasoline savings.
- **Save money.** If you have your menu planned ahead of time, you'll be able to buy the right kind of food in the package size to fit your needs.
- **Save your energy.** Meal planning lends order to time-crunched lives. There's no longer the stress of wondering, "What's for dinner?"

How Do You Plan Menus?

If you are following a meal planning approach, such as the Choose Your Foods: Exchange List for Diabetes, the Diabetes Food Pyramid, or the carbohydrate counting system, you are already off to a great start.

Your meal pattern will tell you which foods you need and how much of each to include. If you are following an exchange/choices diet, you will know how many servings you need from the starch, vegetable, fruit, meat or meat-substitute, milk, and fat lists each day. If you are following the Diabetes Food Pyramid, use the serving guidelines from each section of the pyramid. The carbohydrate counting system outlines the number of grams of carbohydrates you can include at each meal and snack.

No matter what your method of diabetes meal planning, the foods you eat and the timing of your meals should be based on your personal diabetes treatment plan and blood glucose results.

Your meal plan is the basis for your menus and shopping list for the week. An RD can help you develop a meal pattern that is right for you. Having a meal pattern gives you the freedom to decide which foods meet your budget needs.

MEAL PLANNING CHECKLIST

After you try your hand at planning a week's menu, take a moment to review the checklist below.

Do the menus:

✓ follow your individualized diabetes meal plan?

✓ use a variety of foods from all parts of the pyramid?

✓ emphasize nutritious, economical foods?

✓ take advantage of weekly store specials?

✓ include planned-overs?

Use the Ready, Set, Shop! Menus for This Week template on p. 19 to assist in menu planning. The Ready, Set, Shop! Shopping List template on p. 21 can help organize your shopping list for a speedier trip to the market.

To save even more time, keep a master list of all the meals you plan, making it easy to select from these tried-and-true combinations rather than planning new menus every week. You will soon accumulate a large list of economical meals.

PLANNED-OVERS

Leftovers may be your budget's best friend, but no one wants to see the same dish three times in one week. You can save time and money while avoiding mealtime boredom by using planned-overs, foods intentionally left after a meal for use in another meal. Using planned-overs is quite different from reheating yesterday's supper for today's lunch. When you use planned-overs, you are planning ahead for leftovers.

Many of the recipes in this book are designed around the planned-over concept. For example, the chicken left from "Marilyn's Spicy 'Fried' Chicken" (p. 145) is ready for use in "Southwestern Chicken Wrap-Ups" (p. 146). You can plan to use the extra turkey from "Golden Roasted Turkey Breast" (p. 151) in "Tempting Turkey Pot Pie" (p. 152).

If you start thinking about your meals in terms of planned-overs, you'll find easy and interesting examples everywhere. Make a pork roast with vegetables on Sunday, and plan to use the leftover pork later in the week to flavor black beans and rice.

A large round steak in a family pack can provide at least four meals. Cut the steak in half lengthwise, then slice one portion into thin strips (across the grain for tenderness) for use in stir-fry and burritos or fajitas. Freeze the remaining half. You can defrost it at a later date and cube it to make hearty beef stew. If you have scraps left, dice them to use in vegetable beef soup. Be sure to label and date your planned-over foods so that you'll know what you have on hand and use it safely.

NO TIME TO PLAN?

Begin by reviewing the One Week's Sample Menu on pp. 25-29, which can be individualized to suit your needs. These low-cost meals are planned around recipes found in this book. Use the menu as a starting point to plan your week and make a shopping list. If you are still overwhelmed by the thought of planning a week's worth of menus, start by planning five meals.

Planning five meals will take only five minutes—time you can surely find while waiting for a doctor's appointment or for a pot of pasta to boil.

READY, SET, SHOP! MENUS FOR THIS WEEK

Days of the Week	Breakfast	Lunch	Dinner
Sunday			
Monday			
Tuesday			
Wednesday			
Thursday			
Friday			
Saturday			

Cost-Wise Cooking

"I said to my wife, 'Where do you want to go for our anniversary?' She said, 'I want to go somewhere I've never been before.' I said, 'Try the kitchen.'"
—Henny Youngman

Cooking is becoming a lost art, but it is one that you'll need to rediscover if spending less and eating healthfully is your goal. Fast foods and convenience foods do save time, but they are real budget-busters. Don't assume that saving money requires you to become a master chef. Start by looking for recipes like those in this book—quick to assemble, with few ingredients and simple cooking techniques.

Stock Up

Keep your pantry stocked with low cost, healthful grocery staples to save time and trips to the grocery store. With a few basic foods from these parts of the MyPyramid, you'll be ready to cook cost-wise meals in just a few minutes.

- **Grains, beans, and starchy vegetables:** flour, oats, whole-grain breads, cereals, crackers, dry or canned beans, rice, pasta, canned corn, and potatoes.
- **Vegetables:** fresh or plain frozen vegetables, tomato sauce, and canned tomatoes.
- **Fruits:** fresh and plain frozen fruits, fruit canned in juice, applesauce, and frozen concentrated 100% fruit juice.
- **Milk:** fat-free milk, nonfat dry milk, and nonfat yogurt.
- **Meat and others:** chicken, fish, turkey, ground beef, eggs, peanut butter, cheese, and water-packed canned tuna.

You should also have the right kitchen tools on hand to make cooking easier. Important pieces for healthy cooking include a pressure cooker, good-quality sharp knives, a grill, and nonstick cookware. Less expensive tools that should be in your kitchen are a cheese grater, kitchen shears, a steamer basket, a kitchen scale, a cutting board, and a microwave.

READY, SET, SHOP! SHOPPING LIST

Fill out this shopping list and take it with you on your next trip to the grocery store to keep your fridge stocked with all the good-for-you essentials that you need in your diet.

Fresh Vegetables	Fresh Fruit	Bread & Baked Goods
Meat	Dairy	Deli
Canned Vegetables	Canned Fruits	Condiments
Cereals	Baking Goods	Paper Goods
Cleaners	Snacks	Beverages
Pet Care Items	Frozen Foods	Miscellaneous

Now You're Cooking!

Once you're in the kitchen, make the most of your time and money by cooking and baking in large quantities and freezing a portion for future use.

This technique—one way to get planned-overs—is known as batch cooking, and it can be as simple as cooking a few extra chicken breasts to freeze for later use. The idea is to cook once and serve the food two or three times. For example, if you are making pasta at your evening meal, throw some extra noodles in the pot to use in a cold pasta salad for tomorrow's midday meal. Or prepare a large quantity of a standard recipe, such as "Spunky Spaghetti Sauce" (p. 153), to use immediately, then freeze the remainder for use in lasagna or stuffed peppers. Make a large batch of waffles on Sunday morning, serve a few for breakfast, and freeze the rest to pop in the toaster on a busy weekday morning.

You may not have time to cook during the workweek, but you may have some free moments on the weekend to start preparing food for the week ahead. This saves not only time, but also money because you can buy larger amounts of basic ingredients more economically. Make your own healthful microwave meals by separating your planned-overs into microwave-safe dishes in portion sizes that are right for your individual meal plan.

Knowing there's something in your freezer that is just a few microwave minutes away from a meal may be just the incentive you need to skip the expensive fast-food drive-through after work.

Getting the Most From Your Microwave

A microwave is handy for reheating planned-overs, but you can get even more savings from the microwave by using it to:

- Crisp up stale or soggy crackers, cereals, and pretzels. Microwave them in a baking dish on high power until they're very warm (1–3 minutes), stirring once. Let them cool thoroughly to crisp.
- Get more juice from lemons, oranges, and grapefruits. Slice the fruit in half, then microwave it on high power for 30 seconds to 1 minute.
- Extract the last drops from a bottle of pancake syrup. Remove the cap, then microwave the bottle on high power for 20–30 seconds. An empty-looking bottle may hold as much as 1/4 cup of syrup.

Clever, cost-wise cooks know the value of casseroles. These one dish meals can be prepared ahead of time and stored in the refrigerator or freezer, ready to bake at a moment's notice. Casseroles are a great place to use leftover turkey, chicken, beef, rice, and vegetables. This makes for less expensive meals and faster baking. Casseroles can be designed to provide you with foods from each of the food groups in your diabetes meal plan. Take a look at the inexpensive, mix-and-match ingredients in the "Quick Six" casserole plan (pp. 30-31) and invent your own one dish meal.

If you plan to cook your prepared casserole within 24 hours or so, store it raw in the refrigerator and allow about 10–15 minutes of extra oven time to make sure the chilled ingredients are baked through. If you decide to freeze the casserole for future use, wrap the dish securely and freeze it for up to six weeks. Defrost it thoroughly and safely before baking.

SAFETY FIRST

Economical eating requires special attention to food safety, particularly when using planned-overs and storing large amounts of food. For the person with diabetes, the nausea, vomiting, diarrhea, and inability to eat that accompanies foodborne illness are not only unpleasant, but may also have serious effects on blood glucose control.

For safety first in the cost-wise kitchen, pay attention to "sell by" and "use by" dates on the canned, jarred, and packaged foods you purchase. Safe food storage is essential. Store flour and grains in airtight containers and your canned goods in a cool area. Your refrigerator should be set at 40°F or below, while your freezer should be 0°F or colder. When putting away your groceries, keep these additional safety tips in mind:

- Eat canned and jarred goods with a high acid content (tomatoes, grapefruit, and pineapple) within 18 months. Canned foods with a low acid content—meat, poultry, fish, and most vegetables—will keep for 2–5 years.

- Use eggs within three weeks of the expiration date, and keep them refrigerated at all times.

- Refrigerate fresh poultry or fish for no more than two days after you buy it. If it won't be used within two days, freeze it. Other fresh meats will keep in the fridge for up to 3–5 days.

- A food that has been cooked, served, and refrigerated within two hours can be stored safely in the refrigerator for 3–4 days. In the freezer, most planned-overs will store well for 2–3 months.
- When you store planned-overs, divide the food among small containers so that it will cool quickly. Label your storage containers with the food's name and the date it was prepared so that you'll know which items to use first.
- Defrost planned-over batches of frozen foods thoroughly before cooking them. It is best not to go directly from freezer to oven, because bacteria may thrive in the center of a frozen food as the edges begin to cook. It is not safe to defrost food on the kitchen counter at room temperature. Try to plan ahead to thaw your frozen dishes safely in the refrigerator.
- Use your microwave to defrost before cooking only if you will be cooking your dish immediately afterward. Microwave defrosting often cooks parts of the food, and storing partly cooked food can lead to bacteria buildup.

BAGGING THE BARGAIN:
One Week's Sample Menus for $7 a Day—or Less!

DAY 1 (4.19)
Breakfast
1 cup sliced strawberries ($0.84)
1 6-oz container no sugar added, fat-free yogurt ($0.40)
2 Golden Applesauce Muffins ($0.24)*
1 cup hot tea ($0.04)

Lunch
2 cups Favorite Vegetable Soup ($0.90)*
6 saltine crackers ($0.06)
1/2 medium banana ($0.04)
1 cup fat-free milk ($0.16)

Dinner
1 Grilled Asian Pork Kabob ($0.98)*
1 cup Crunchy Oriental Coleslaw ($0.22)*
1 serving Rich Chocolate Fudge Cake ($0.17)*
12 oz iced tea ($0.04)

Snack
3/4 oz pretzels (about 7–8 large pretzel twists) ($0.06)
8 oz sugar-free lemonade ($0.04)

DAY 2 ($3.61)
Breakfast
1 serving Hearty Oatmeal for One ($0.64)*
1 cup fat-free milk ($0.16)

Lunch
2/3 cup cooked spaghetti noodles ($0.04)
1/2 cup Spunky Spaghetti Sauce ($0.44)*
1 serving Quick Garlic Buns ($0.06)*
2 cups chopped lettuce & tomato ($0.48)
1 Tbsp olive oil and vinegar ($0.06)
1 Chocolate Peanut Butter Drop ($0.06)*
12 oz iced tea ($0.04)

Dinner

3 oz Golden Roasted Turkey Breast ($0.37)*
1 cup Carrots, Onions, and Potatoes ($0.30)*
1/2 cup Southern-Style Green Beans ($0.25)*
1 roll ($0.11)
1 tsp light margarine ($0.01)
1 Pumpkin Bar ($0.13)*
1 cup fat-free milk ($0.16)

Snack

1 medium apple ($0.30)

DAY 3 ($5.48)

Breakfast

1 scrambled egg ($0.06)
2 slices whole-wheat toast ($0.10)
2 tsp light margarine ($0.02)
2 tsp 100% fruit spread ($0.09)
1 cup Berry and Banana Blend ($0.61)*

Lunch (Fast Food)

1 small chili with 4 crackers ($0.99)
1 side salad with 1 packet light dressing ($0.99)
1 small diet soda ($1.09)

Dinner

1 cup Sunday Afternoon Split Pea Soup ($0.29)*
1 serving Gran's Country-Style Corn Bread ($0.08)*
1 Personal Fruit Parfait ($0.77)*
1 cup fat-free milk ($0.16)

Snack

3 cups air-popped popcorn ($0.04) with
2 tsp light margarine, melted ($0.02)
12 oz diet soda ($0.17)

DAY 4 ($4.46)

Breakfast

3/4 cup bran flake cereal ($0.06) with
1/2 cup fat-free milk ($0.08)
1 English muffin ($0.17) with
2 tsp reduced-calorie margarine ($0.02) and
2 tsp 100% fruit spread ($0.09)
1 cup coffee ($0.04)

Lunch

1 turkey sandwich: 2 oz leftover Golden Roasted Turkey Breast*
on 2 slices whole-wheat bread with 1 tsp mustard ($0.35)
1/2 cup Sassy Sweet Potato Chips ($0.16)*
1 cup carrot and celery sticks ($0.10) with
2 Tbsp fat-free ranch-style dressing ($0.12)
1 medium apple ($0.30)
12 oz diet soda ($0.17)

Dinner

1 serving Beef and Broccoli Stroganoff ($1.69)*
Sliced tomato and cucumber (1/2 small tomato,
1/4 medium cucumber) ($0.24) with
1 Tbsp Versatile Vinaigrette ($0.12)*
1 slice French bread ($0.06) with
1 tsp reduced-calorie margarine ($0.01)
1 Rainbow Parfait ($0.40)*
12 oz iced tea ($0.04)

Snack

1/2 cup fat-free, sugar-free chocolate pudding ($0.24)

DAY 5 ($3.64)

Breakfast

1 slice Cinnamon French Toast ($0.07)*
1 tsp light margarine ($0.01)
1 Tbsp maple syrup ($0.05)
2 slices turkey bacon ($0.16)
1/2 cup unsweetened apple juice ($0.06)

Lunch

1 Gourmet Grilled Cheese Sandwich ($0.72)*
1 oz baked tortilla chips ($0.28)
1/2 cup mandarin oranges canned in juice ($0.16)
12 oz diet soda ($0.17)

Dinner

1 serving Marilyn's Spicy "Fried" Chicken ($0.50)*
1 serving Green Bean Stir-Fry ($0.48)*
1 medium ear corn on the cob ($0.22) with
1 tsp light margarine ($0.01)
1 serving Spiced Raisin Bread Pudding ($0.23)*
12 oz iced tea ($0.04)

Snack

1 cup Do-It-Yourself Drinkable Yogurt ($0.48)*

DAY 6 ($3.75)

Breakfast

1/2 cup unsweetened pineapple juice ($0.20)
1 serving Cinnamon Coffeecake ($0.28)*
1 cup fat-free milk ($0.16)

Lunch

1 Southwestern Chicken Wrap-Up ($0.38)*
1 medium pear ($0.43)
1 cup Apple-Raspberry Tea Sparkler ($0.18)*

Dinner

3 oz Seasoned Pan-Fried Catfish ($0.80)*
1/2 cup Crunchy Oriental Coleslaw ($0.11)*
1/2 cup Garden Vegetable Scramble ($0.46)*
1 roll ($0.11) with
1 tsp reduced-calorie margarine ($0.01)
1 serving Simple Strawberry Shortcake ($0.35)*

Snack

1 leftover Golden Applesauce Muffin ($0.12)*
1 cup fat-free milk ($0.16)

DAY 7 ($3.79)

Breakfast
1 cup tomato juice ($0.30)
1 serving Eggs in a Basket ($0.16)*
2 slices turkey bacon ($0.16)

Lunch
1 cup leftover Sunday Afternoon Split Pea Soup ($0.29)*
6 saltine crackers ($0.06)
1 slice fat-free American cheese ($0.15)
1 serving leftover Simple Strawberry Shortcake ($0.35)*
1 cup fat-free milk ($0.16)

Dinner
1 1/2 cups Tempting Turkey Pot Pie ($0.64)*
2 cups lettuce, tomato, cucumber, and carrot salad ($0.48)
2 tablespoons Versatile Vinaigrette ($0.24)*
1 Banana-Split Parfait ($0.60)*
12 oz iced tea ($0.04)

Snack
1 cup Tropical Slushy ($0.16)*

*Recipe included in this book.

The "Quick Six" Casserole Plan

Looking for a quick and easy way to plan an inexpensive, yet healthful meal? Use the "Quick Six" casserole plan, a way to mix and match basic ingredients for added variety and economical eating. Ideas range from a classic chicken casserole built around chicken soup, broccoli, rice, chicken, Parmesan cheese, and bread crumbs to a vegetarian casserole made from Italian-style diced tomatoes, yellow squash, olives, celery, bell pepper, garlic, and mozzarella cheese.

1. Choose one sauce-maker
   1 can (10 3/4 oz) reduced-fat cream of mushroom soup, undiluted
   1 can (10 3/4 oz) reduced-fat cream of celery soup, undiluted
   1 can (10 3/4 oz) reduced-fat cream of chicken soup, undiluted
   1 can (10 3/4 oz) cheddar cheese soup, undiluted
   1 can (10 3/4 oz) cream of potato soup, undiluted
   2 cans (14 3/4 oz) Italian-style diced tomatoes, drained

2. Choose one frozen vegetable
   1 package (10 oz) frozen chopped spinach, thawed
   1 package (10 oz) frozen cut broccoli, thawed
   1 package (10 oz) frozen French-style green beans, thawed
   1 package (10 oz) frozen peas, thawed
   1 package (16 oz) frozen sliced yellow squash, thawed
   1 package (10 oz) frozen whole kernel corn, thawed
   1 package (10 oz) frozen mixed vegetables, thawed

3. Choose one pasta/rice/potato
   2 cups cooked elbow macaroni
   1 cup uncooked rice
   4 cups uncooked cholesterol-free wide egg noodles
   3 cups uncooked medium pasta shells
   3 cups frozen shredded hash brown potatoes, thawed

4. Choose one meat/fish/poultry
   2 cans (6 oz each) water-packed solid white tuna, drained and flaked
   2 cups chopped cooked chicken
   2 cups chopped cooked ham
   2 cups chopped cooked turkey
   1 lb lean ground turkey or beef, browned and drained

5. Choose one or more extras (optional)

1 can (4 oz) sliced mushrooms, drained
1/2 cup sliced ripe olives
1/4 cup chopped bell pepper
1/4 cup chopped onion
1/2 cup chopped celery
1/4 cup shredded carrot
2 garlic cloves, minced
1 can (4 1/2 oz) chopped green chili peppers
1 package (1 1/4 oz) taco seasoning mix

6. Choose one or two toppings

1/2 cup (2 oz) shredded 2% milk reduced-fat mozzarella cheese
1/2 cup grated Parmesan cheese
1/2 cup (2 oz) shredded low-fat Swiss cheese
1/2 cup (2 oz) shredded low-fat cheddar cheese
1/2 cup fine, dry breadcrumbs
1/2 cup dry stuffing mix
1/2 cup crushed cornflake cereal

Combine one sauce-maker with 1 cup low-fat sour cream, 1 cup low-fat milk, 1 cup water, 1 tsp salt, and 1 tsp pepper (omit sour cream and milk when using tomatoes). Stir in the frozen vegetable, pasta/rice/potato, meat/fish/poultry, and any extras. Spoon the mixture into a 9 × 13-inch baking dish coated with cooking spray. Sprinkle with a topping. Bake the casserole covered at 350°F for 1 hour and 10 minutes. Uncover and bake for 10 more minutes or until bubbly. Yield: 12 servings.

Money $aving Tip

To save yourself more money, recycle the plastic plates from commercial microwaveable frozen dinners to use for preparing your meals.

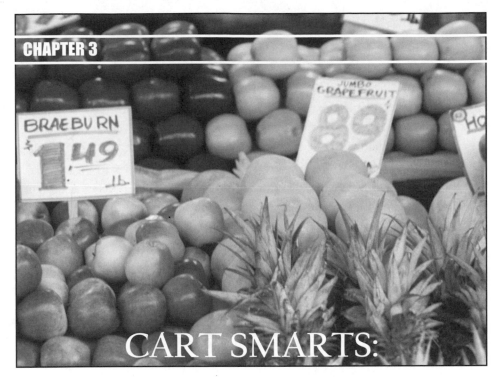

CHAPTER 3

CART SMARTS:

SHOPPING TO WIN
THE GROCERY STORE GAME

The typical American household spends almost 14 cents of every dollar it earns on food. Although a portion of the money is spent on food eaten away from home, savvy supermarket shopping is one sure way to spend less and eat healthfully.

Your choice of a shopping site depends on your time and saving priorities. The smartest shoppers often visit a combination of markets: the warehouse club once a month to stock up on nonperishable staples in large sizes, the supercenter to find the best everyday prices, and the regular supermarket to save time.

Supermarkets are case studies in smart selling. In fact, grocery carts were invented because customers had a tendency to stop shopping when their baskets became too full or too heavy. This chapter will help you win the grocery store game by outlining simple shopping strategies to slash your grocery bill.

Shopping for a Supermarket

The corner market is no longer the only place to spend your food dollars. Location and convenience are important factors in selecting a store because most of us visit our supermarket at least once a week. However, it pays to know about the other options in the marketplace so that you can choose the one that offers you the most savings, based on your shopping style and priorities.

Once you select your shopping site, join the shoppers' club if your store has one. As a member, you'll receive a card that entitles you to automatic discounts or access to unadvertised, members-only specials.

Food Co-op

A food co-op is one option for near-wholesale prices on grains, beans, and other bulk foods. But regular supermarkets, supercenters, and warehouse clubs are more commonly available.

Regular Supermarket

The regular supermarket is the choice of almost 85% of shoppers. Everyday prices may be higher than at larger superstores, but specials and store brands are abundant. The supermarket's smaller scale means faster shopping. That can save both time and money because more time in the grocery store usually adds up to a larger grocery bill. Research from the Food Marketing Institute shows that shoppers spend close to $2 for every extra minute in the market.

Supercenter

The supercenter combines a grocery store, a pharmacy, a florist, and other merchandise under one huge roof—they're often the size of six or seven typical supermarkets. Supercenters have a tremendous selection of items in most grocery categories. They tend to have low everyday prices and may even offer to match the weekly specials found in regular supermarkets.

Supercenters have many price advantages because of their size, but shopping in them is more time-consuming and challenging. Because they must be built on a large plot of undeveloped land, they are often located away from residential neighborhoods.

Warehouse Club

The warehouse club is a no-frills approach to food shopping. It offers minimal service, with few advertisements and a stark shopping environment. It typically charges an annual membership fee (although many provide a free one day pass). While the supercenter offers a wide variety of items, the warehouse club has few choices of brands or sizes within brands. Shoppers are offered mass quantities of food, such as 5-pound boxes of crackers or cases of canned pears, at low prices. This may be a good way to stock up on staples if you have the storage space. However, a gallon tub of mayonnaise is not a good buy if it spoils before you can use it all.

What will food shoppers face in the future? In addition to the now-familiar self-checkout kiosks, a number of supermarkets are testing high-tech gadgets such as a combination hand-held barcode reader and wireless shopping cart computer that enables a shopper to scan groceries as they are placed in the cart while the computer keeps a running tally of purchases, offering appropriate instant discount coupons for items right on the spot. Kiosks next to the deli counter let customers preorder their deli items and pick them up later. By making shopping faster and easier, supermarket operators hope to build customer loyalty.

SHOPPING FOR SINGLES

According to the most recent U.S. Census information, almost 10% of the country's total population lives alone. Here are some tips for single shoppers to maximize food dollars at the grocery store:

- Buy frozen fruit and vegetables in bags so you can use only what you need and freeze the rest.
- Look for foods sold in single servings, such as juice, yogurt, frozen meals, soup, and pudding. Better yet, buy the lower priced larger versions and make your own single-serving items.
- Shopping from the bulk bins will enable you to buy smaller amounts.
- The butcher or produce manager can assist you by packaging smaller amounts of prepackaged items.
- Produce that keeps longer in the refrigerator may be a good choice: broccoli, Brussels sprouts, cabbage, and carrots.
- When you buy a loaf of bread, take out what you'll need for the week, then wrap and freeze the rest.

How Does Your Shopping Stack Up?

Take this quick quiz to determine if you're a savvy shopper!

1. Do you shop alone?
The more the merrier....except in the grocery store. Shopping with extra people means extra food in the cart and extra dollars spent at checkout. Consumers who shop alone are more likely to stick with their shopping list.

2. Do you shop when you're hungry?
Rather than being inspired, you could find yourself tossing an extra snack or two into the grocery basket if you're famished. A small snack before you shop may help avoid temptation.

3. What time of day do you shop?
Shop early in the day if you can. Tired shoppers are more inclined to buy on impulse and make poor food choices. Set a routine. Establish a day and time when it is easy for you to move quickly through the store, staying focused on your shopping needs.

4. Do you shop from a list?
Planning your meals for the week and writing a list of ingredients you need will make it possible for you to avoid buying costly impulse items. Use the "Ready, Set, Shop! Shopping List" on p. 21 to organize your next shopping expedition.

5. Do you buy generic store brands?
Grocery stores often obtain their generic brands from exactly the same manufacturer of their regular brands. You can save at least $0.20 to $0.30 for every dollar you spend on generic versions of store brand products.

Don't Leave Home Without It

Don't leave home for a shopping trip without planning. The smartest shoppers shrink grocery bills before they even set foot in the store.

Make a Plan

Use the tips in Chapter 2 to plan your menus for the week based on what you already have on hand, leftovers, sales, and coupon/rebate items. Minimize the number of trips you make to the store each week.

Neatness Counts

Keep your refrigerator, freezer, and cabinets organized so you don't buy food you already have.

Be a List Lover

Plan your shopping trip by making a list of what you'll need for the week's menu and stick with it! If you shop without a list, you are more apt to make impulse buys. Picking up an extra two or three items on a shopping trip can add up to $5 to $10 a week—that's $260 to $520 a year in extra spending!

To save minutes as well as money, organize your list to match the aisle-by-aisle layout of your favorite grocery store. Research shows that the more efficiently you make your way through the store, the less you'll spend.

Check Out the Specials

Supermarkets frequently offer "loss leaders." These are heavily advertised low-profit items designed to lure you into the store. Check store ads and fliers for sales and specials. Keep a price notebook listing the items you buy regularly and their typical prices. Note what's on sale. Your notes will serve as a guide to the week's best buys.

Shopping the specials doesn't require spending hours traveling to several stores each week. You'll find that many stores have predictable sale cycles. For example, you may be able to stock up on canned goods or boneless chicken breasts every six weeks, when your supermarket of choice offers them for sale.

Cut Costs With Coupons

Coupons are money-savers if you use them on items that you normally buy. With planning, coupons can save you on average between $5 and $20 for every $100 you spend on groceries. However, less than 3% of all coupons issued are redeemed. On shopping day, select the coupons you'll need and attach them to your list. Don't forget: Many stores now have instant coupon dispensers within reach of the products being discounted.

Double up on value

Use coupons in combination with store sales and double/triple coupon days. Coupons don't always guarantee the best bargain, however, many times it is still less expensive to purchase the store brand of an item than to buy a brand name with a coupon. Shop carefully.

Although the money saved by clipping coupons may not seem like much, it does add up. Using just five coupons a week at $0.50 each means a savings of $130 a year. If you need additional positive reinforcement for the time and effort it takes to clip coupons, review your weekly cash register receipts and stash the money you saved using coupons into a jar. Put aside that cash for a special treat for yourself or your family.

Ask and you shall receive

If you like a particular product, call the toll-free consumer center number listed on its package. You'll often receive coupons for that item if you ask. Also, request that your local store start holding double or triple coupon days. If a sale item is sold out, ask for a rain check. Stores are required by law to provide a rain check so that you can buy the item at the sale price the next time you visit.

WHAT'S IN STORE?

It's time for your supermarket safari. Venture ahead only if you are in the proper frame of mind—it's a jungle out there! Along with your shopping list, you may want to take a tape player or radio with headphones to listen to some fast-paced music while you shop. Supermarkets often play soft, soothing music to encourage you to shop slowly and therefore spend more money. Research indicates that listening to upbeat music will get you out of the store faster, lowering your grocery bill.

Basket, Please

If you only need a few items, grab a basket instead of a cart. A spacious cart gives you the feeling that you need to buy more, while a small basket helps you stick to your short list because you'll be ready to leave when it gets heavy.

Shop With Your Eyes Wide Open

Smart shoppers are aware of the marketing strategies used in the grocery store. Stores are designed so that the high-traffic areas, such as the dairy and meat departments, are in the back. This means you'll have to pass through more aisles to reach them and are more likely to pick up a few extra things on the way.

Foods that go together—chips, dips, and soft drinks—are often grouped together to encourage impulse buys. Another market strategy is to place a basic food item, such as cereal, across the aisle from an impulse item, like candy. Cartons of merchandise stacked in the aisles also slow you down and suggest bargain pricing. Compare prices carefully before buying.

Grocers place the most expensive brands and impulse items at eye level. You'll have to look on high and low shelves to find the best buys. Beware of bargains that aren't really bargains. Signs saying "new" or "special" may catch your eye, but they do not necessarily point out low-priced items.

Location, Location, Location

Often, the same or similar items are sold at different prices in different parts of the store. Imported Swiss cheese at the deli counter may cost 25% more than the prepackaged store brand Swiss cheese in the dairy case. Sodas are another case in point. A 20-oz bottle of a diet soft drink may cost $0.99 if purchased at the small refrigerator case at the checkout counter, while a much larger, 2-liter bottle in the soft drink aisle may cost you as little as $0.89.

Don't Be Snobby About Store Brands

Store brands or private-label items are often priced as much as 30% below their national-brand competitors. Most shoppers find store brands taste as good as brand names. Not surprisingly, brand-name manufacturers often make the same exact items for the supermarket brands.

Reading Food Labels

Use the unit price to compare the costs of different brands and package sizes. Unit price is the price per ounce, pound, or pint. Most stores show the unit price on the display shelf. Read nutrition information labels too. (See "Label Reading 101" on p. 42.) The ingredient list can reveal important health information as well. The ingredients are listed in order from most to least amount found in the product. Avoid buying foods with empty calorie ingredients listed as the first or second item on the list.

Compare Cost per Edible Serving

Compare the costs per servings of different varieties of meats, fresh fruits, and vegetables. The price per pound is not always a good basis for comparing the costs of these foods because of the varying amounts of bones, fat, cores, pits, skins, and other parts you can't eat. For example, after cooking, you can get 3, 3-oz servings of lean meat per pound from an item with little or no fat or bone, such as round steak. However, you'll only get one serving of lean meat per pound from an item with a greater amount of bone, gristle, and fat, like spareribs.

BEST BUYS, BAD BUYS

Best Buys

- Nonfat dry milk for baking and cooking
- Popcorn kernels to air pop for snacks
- Large bags of plain, frozen vegetables
- Bags of dry beans
- Regular or quick-cooking oats

Bad Buys

- Individually wrapped, single-serving packages
- Giant boxes of low-nutrient foods
- Vegetables frozen with seasonings and sauces
- Deli meats—bake a small turkey/ham and slice it for sandwiches
- Microwaveable breakfasts

Is Bigger Better?

Buy economy-sized items only if you have space for storage and you can use them before they spoil. Large packages may not always be a better buy, particularly when a smaller-sized item has been specially priced. Also, buying in bulk may bulk you up. Studies show that people tend to eat more at each sitting when they have access to especially large packages of food.

Skip the "Special" Food

People with diabetes don't require special diabetic foods. Although these products may be convenient, they are high priced. Eat healthy foods at healthy prices, while keeping an eye on nutrient content and portion size.

Money-Saving Markdowns

You can save money by purchasing products that are discounted in special sale carts or damaged product bins. Check the items first for freshness and package condition and pay close attention to the expiration dates. You may be pouring money down the drain if you buy a gallon of milk just before it expires. Shop Sunday morning for bargains on high-priced meats, such as chicken cordon bleu and stuffed veal. Because these meats are more perishable than plain meats, stores discount them in the morning to sell quickly.

What's the Price of Convenience?

If it's been grated, chopped, precooked, presliced, or individually packaged, you may be paying the price for convenience. However, convenience can pay off. For example, if you only need a handful of broccoli florets for a salad, buy them from the supermarket salad bar instead of purchasing the entire head of broccoli.

The premium you pay for buying salad that's washed, chopped, and bagged varies by the type of salad you're buying. A common salad of iceberg lettuce, cabbage, and carrots costs about the same whether homemade or prepackaged. A salad of more exotic Italian-style greens, such as romaine lettuce and radicchio, costs more than twice as much if prepackaged.

Be Flexible

Although your list is your lifeline, take advantage of in-store specials by substituting them for similar foods in your meal plan. If you planned to buy grapes but find that apples are on sale, make the switch to save more.

At the Checkout Counter

You're almost out the door, but don't forget to use the checkout counter as a last chance for additional savings opportunities. Although the accuracy rate is usually high, supermarket scanner errors can cost you money. Make sure to check your receipt before leaving the store; many supermarket chains will give you the item free if the wrong price is scanned. Find out your store's policy for pricing mistakes. Also, if you pay for groceries with a debit card or a check, ask for extra cash back to save yourself a trip to the bank—and the fee that bank machines often charge.

LABEL READING 101

Nutrition Facts

Serving Size 1 cup (228g)
Servings Per Container 2

Amount Per Serving

Calories 260	Calories from Fat 120

	% Daily Value*
Total Fat 13g	**20%**
Saturated Fat 5g	**25%**
Trans Fat 2g	
Cholesterol 30mg	**10%**
Sodium 660mg	**28%**
Total Carbohydrate 31g	**10%**
Dietary Fiber 0g	**0%**
Sugars 5g	
Protein 5g	

Vitamin A 4%	•	Vitamin C 2%
Calcium 15%	•	Iron 4%

* Percent Daily Values are based on a 2,000 calorie diet. Your Daily Values may be higher or lower depending on your calorie needs.

	Calories:	2,000	2,500
Total Fat	Less than	65g	80g
Sat Fat	Less than	20g	25g
Cholesterol	Less than	300mg	300mg
Sodium	Less than	2,400mg	2,400mg
Total Carbohydrate		300g	375g
Dietary Fiber		25g	30g

Calories per gram:

Fat 9   •   Carbohydrate 4   •   Protein 4

Careful label reading is the best bet to ensure that you get the most for your nutrition dollar. The Nutrition Facts label lists what are known as Daily Values, which tell you how much of each nutrient should be eaten in a day. Daily Values for a 2,000-calorie diet are printed on food labels, but your own nutrition needs may be higher or lower than the numbers on the label. Consult an RD for help with interpreting food labels to meet your individual nutrition needs.

The FDA now allows manufacturers to make certain claims linking the effect of a nutrient or a food to a disease or a health-related condition. Only claims supported by scientific evidence are allowed. The food used in the claim must be an adequate source of the appropriate nutrients.

Two claims related to heart disease are of particular interest to people with diabetes:

- A diet low in saturated fat and cholesterol may help reduce the risk of coronary heart disease.
- A diet rich in fruits, vegetables, and grain products that contain fiber, particularly soluble fiber, and are low in saturated fat and cholesterol may help reduce the risk of coronary heart disease.

Reading Between the Lines

The following key terms have been defined by the FDA and are commonly found on food labels on grocery store shelves:

"Free" means that a product contains none of the designated ingredient or only amounts that would not significantly affect the body.

- **Calorie Free:** Less than 5 calories per serving
- **Cholesterol Free:** Less than 2 mg of cholesterol per serving and 2 grams or less of saturated fat per serving
- **Fat Free:** Less than 0.5 grams of fat per serving
- **Saturated Fat Free:** Less than 0.5 grams of saturated fat and 0.5 grams of trans fatty acids per serving
- **Sodium Free:** Less than 5 mg of sodium per serving
- **Sugar Free:** Less than 0.5 grams of sugar per serving
- **Zero G Trans Fat:** Less than 0.5 grams of trans fatty acids per serving

"Low" may be used on foods that can be eaten often without exceeding the USDA/HHS dietary guidelines. Note that "low carb" has not yet been defined by the FDA.

- **Low Calorie:** 40 calories or less per serving
- **Low Cholesterol:** 20 mg or less of cholesterol per serving and 2 grams or less of saturated fat per serving
- **Low Fat:** 3 grams or less of fat per serving
- **Low Saturated Fat:** 1 gram or less of saturated fat per serving and 15% or less of calories from saturated fat
- **Low Sodium:** 140 mg or less of sodium per serving

"Reduced" means that the product has been changed nutritionally and now contains at least 25% less of a given nutrient or 25% fewer calories than the regular version. However, if a product is already naturally low in that nutrient, such as peanut butter—which is already low in cholesterol—the label can't claim that it is "reduced."

"High" means that the food contains 20% or more of the Daily Value for a particular nutrient per serving.

"Good" source means that one serving of the food contains 10–19% of the Daily Value for a particular nutrient per serving.

"Light" has more than one meaning. A product is "light" if it contains 1/3 fewer calories or 1/2 the fat of the regular product. It can also mean that the sodium content of a low-calorie, low-fat food has been reduced by at least 50%. Finally, "light" can simply describe the product's texture and color.

"Healthy" on a label means that the food must be low in unsaturated and saturated fats and contain specific amounts of cholesterol, sodium, and other vitamins and minerals.

"Lean" describes the fat content of meat, poultry, and seafood. A product is considered lean when it contains less than 10 grams of total fat, 4.5 grams or less of saturated fat, and less than 95 mg of cholesterol per 3-oz serving.

"Fresh" means the food is raw, has never been frozen or heated, and contains no preservatives. Fresh frozen can be used for foods that are quickly frozen while still fresh.

Money $aving Tip
- Take the time to mail in rebate and refund offers
- Trade coupons with friends
- Clip coupons and organize them by supermarket aisle

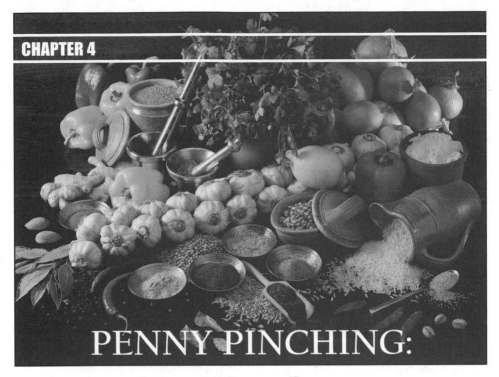

CHAPTER 4

PENNY PINCHING:

The Cost-Wary Consumer's Food Pyramid

Eating right is an investment in your health. The better care you take of your body, the less often you'll need to visit your health care professional. The amount of money you spend on nutritious groceries is very small compared to today's rising medical costs.

As you learned in Chapter 1, people with diabetes don't require expensive special foods or exotic ingredients to meet their nutrition goals. To stay healthy, you need to eat the proper amount of each type of food every day. Following the USDA Food Guide MyPyramid or the Diabetes Food Pyramid will help you make the food choices that are essential to your diabetes care. Both are guides to good eating, however, the Diabetes Food Pyramid is more focused on diabetes meal planning than the MyPyramid.

This chapter is a guide to penny pinching and best buys in all sections of the food pyramid as it appears in the American Diabetes Association's, *The First Step in Diabetes Meal Planning*. Grab your grocery cart and calculator and start saving.

GRAINS, BEANS, AND STARCHY VEGETABLES

The foods in this group are the foundation of an inexpensive, healthy meal plan. They are low in cost, low in fat (unless prepared with added fat), and generally high in fiber. Eat six or more servings from this group every day, depending on your specific meal plan.

BEST BUYS

- Cornmeal
- Flour
- Farina
- Grits
- Ready-to-eat cereals, such as corn, wheat, and bran flakes; puffed rice and oat cereals; and shredded wheat
- Rolled oats
- Bread
- Hamburger or hot dog buns
- Saltines
- Popcorn kernels
- Dry beans
- Rice
- Pasta
- Corn
- Potatoes
- Sweet potatoes and yams, fresh

$$ Thrifty Tips $$

$ Buy unsweetened cereal in bags rather than boxes. Packaging costs money.

$ Try generic or store-brand cereals to save 20–30% over the cost of brand name cereals. If you find it hard to make the switch, mix a generic cereal with a brand name of the same type to extend your savings.

$ Stay away from single-serving packets or boxes of cereals.

$ Cook your own hot cereal to save money. Regular or quick-cooking oats are much less expensive than instant oats.

$ Purchase lower priced day-old bread to use for breadcrumbs, French toast, croutons, stuffing, and bread pudding. Even though it may be a bit stale, day-old pound cake is fine to use for a layered fruit trifle dessert.

$ Rolls made from a mix or from dough found in the dairy case are cheaper and tastier than packaged or bakery rolls.

$ Instead of an expensive ready-made pizza crust, buy frozen bread dough, thaw it, and roll it out for a low-cost pizzeria taste.

$ Dry beans triple in volume when they're soaked and cooked. A 1-pound bag will make six 1-cup servings.

$ Blended bean mixes and gourmet beans are almost three times as expensive as bean mixes you make yourself.

$ Canned and frozen beans are good buys, and they save you time as well.

$ Instant, quick-cooking, and seasoned rice mixes cost almost three times more than plain rice that you cook and season yourself.

$ For convenience, buy regular rice, cook more than you need, and freeze the extra for future use.

$ Pasta is cheaper when purchased in bags rather than boxes.

$ Pasta shapes are interchangeable in recipes. Choose the least expensive pasta and substitute it for a more expensive variety of a similar size and shape:
  - Long, thin noodles: fettuccine, linguine, spaghetti, spaghettini, or vermicelli
  - Twisted and curved pasta: cavatappi, elbow macaroni, farfalle, fusilli, orecchiette, radiatore, rotelle, or seashell macaroni
  - Tube-shaped pasta: mostaccioli, penne, rigatoni, or ziti
  - Small tube- or rice-shaped pasta: orzo, or tubetti

$ Compare the prices of different forms of the same starchy vegetable. If you plan to mash sweet potatoes and the price for fresh is almost the same as the price for canned, buy the canned sweet potatoes. They will require less preparation time for you, and you won't be paying for the peelings.

$ Check the drained weight of a can of corn. Frozen corn may be more economical.

$ Potatoes are less expensive if purchased in 10-pound bags.

VEGETABLES

Vegetables are naturally low in fat and calories and are a great source of vitamins and minerals. Eat at least 3–5 servings per day, according to your specific meal plan.

BEST BUYS

- Bean sprouts
- Green beans, fresh
- Onions
- Sauerkraut
- Carrots
- Lettuce
- Turnip greens, canned
- Celery
- Tomatoes, canned
- Mustard greens
- Kale
- Cabbage
- Cucumbers

$$ Thrifty Tips $$

$ Simpler is smarter. Vegetables frozen in butter sauce cost twice as much as plain frozen vegetables—and they have more calories.

$ If you are purchasing bagged fresh vegetables, weigh a few bags and choose the heaviest. There may be as much as a 3/4-pound difference between two 5-pound bags of onions.

$ Use marked-down vegetables for soups, stews, and stir-fry.

$ If the cost of lettuce is too high, use cabbage or other leafy greens (such as kale, spinach, and Swiss chard) to make salads.

$ When buying fresh greens by weight, be sure to shake off the excess water before you put them in your cart. It's amazing how much water can be hidden in the leaves.

$ Bagged, fresh spinach will give you more for your money because it contains fewer stems.

$ Be careful about spending extra money on organic vegetables. You may be paying more than you need to.

$ Fresh vegetables "in season" are a best buy. You may want to buy extras and freeze them to use throughout the year. Economical and nutritious choices in the winter include turnips, carrots, and cabbage.

$ If fresh vegetables are too expensive, use frozen or canned. Pour just the amount you need from a 1-pound bag of frozen vegetables, then twist tie and refreeze the remainder for later use. Although higher in sodium, canned vegetables contain the same nutritional value and may be lower priced. If sodium is a concern, rinse and drain the vegetables before using them, but keep in mind that you may be rinsing away some nutrients.

$ Make your own tomato sauce and save. Just simmer canned tomatoes with green peppers, onions, and spices until thick.

$ Convenience costs money. One pound of carrots may cost about $1.29, but a bag of preshredded carrots may be priced at $1.39 for 10 oz—almost $2.24 per pound. Consider the so-called "baby carrots," which cost $1.99 per pound. Mini carrots are actually regular-sized carrots processed in a tumbler. You pay for the convenience of having them peeled and cut to a suitable size. Make your own mini carrot sticks, saving money and keeping them fresh longer while preserving their nutrition.

$ Remember to consider the edible weight of vegetables. Different vegetables yield a different number of servings per pound; for example, 5–6 servings per pound of green beans, 4–5 servings per pound of Brussels sprouts, and 3–4 servings per pound of broccoli.

$ For the most economical vegetables, grow your own! See Chapter 5.

FRUITS

Fruits are a good source of vitamins, minerals, and fiber. They are sweet tasting and fat free—a winning combination when a snack attack hits. Eat at least 2–4 servings daily, according to your individual meal plan.

BEST BUYS	
■ Apples	■ Grapefruit
■ Oranges	■ Tangerines
■ Pears, fresh	■ Fruit juices, including orange,
■ Applesauce	grapefruit, apple, grape,
■ Bananas	pineapple, and prune

$$ Thrifty Tips $$

$ Apples and oranges cost less when bought by the bag rather than individually. Snack on the perfect pieces and use the less-than-perfect ones for apple crisp or fruit salad.

$ Fresh fruits "in season" are a good buy. Economical choices are apples, pears, bananas, and citrus fruits—oranges, grapefruits, and tangerines.

$ If fresh fruit is too expensive, buy frozen or canned fruit. Rinse syrup off canned fruits if you are concerned about carbohydrate content.

$ Buy fresh berries on sale. Freeze them on a cookie sheet, and then store them in plastic bags in the freezer to use year-round.

$ Price fruits with an eye to the cost per edible serving. If you are paying by the pound, you will be paying for the inedible seeds and rind.

$ Avoid shopping for produce on Sunday evening, when stock is low and the new bounty has yet to arrive. It may be possible to negotiate a discount on bruised fruits and vegetables if you speak with the produce manager.

$ Think twice about buying expensive "organically grown" fruits, even though organic fruits are cleaner, safer, and closer to nature.

$ Frozen concentrated juice is a better buy than cartons or jars of reconstituted juice or juice boxes.

$ Mix canned fruit with fresh seasonal fruit for a low-cost fruit cup.

Milk

Dive into dairy foods, such as milk and yogurt, for a rich source of calcium and many vitamins and minerals. Select 2–3 servings a day from the dairy group, depending on your specific meal plan.

Best Buys

- Fat-free milk
- Plain yogurt
- Nonfat dry milk
- Evaporated milk

$$ Thrifty Tips $$

$ Use nonfat dry milk for drinking, cooking, and baking. It is inexpensive and has a long shelf life. When using nonfat dry milk for a beverage, mix it several hours ahead and refrigerate it so it will be icy cold before you pour a glass.

$ Although you shouldn't buy more milk than you can safely use before the expiration date, a gallon is usually more economical than a quart or a half gallon. Check the unit price to be sure. Also, try to find a gallon with the longest period before expiration.

$ If you only need a small amount of buttermilk in a recipe, don't bother buying an entire quart. You can make "sour" milk by stirring 1 Tbsp of lemon juice or vinegar into enough milk to equal 1 cup. Let the mixture stand for 5 minutes, then use it the same as you would buttermilk.

$ Instead of buying small containers of yogurt, buy a quart and separate it into 1-cup servings yourself.

$ Make fruit or flavored yogurt by adding your own fruit to plain yogurt. It's a better buy and better nutrition.

$ Substitute canned evaporated milk for more expensive whipped cream in an aerosol can. Whip the evaporated milk yourself using an ice-cold bowl and an electric mixer.

MEAT AND OTHERS

Americans spend a significant amount of every food dollar on meat, so considerable food savings can be found in this part of the pyramid. In the Diabetes Food Pyramid, this group contains various types of meats, along with other protein foods—such as cheese, seafood, eggs, and peanut butter. Two to three servings of 2–3 oz each are recommended every day as a good source of protein and certain vitamins and minerals.

BEST BUYS	
■ Ground beef	■ Dry beans
■ Beef chuck roast	■ Eggs
■ Beef chuck steak	■ Peanut butter
■ Fresh pork: Boston butt and shoulder	■ Tuna, canned
	■ Pasteurized processed cheese
■ Cured pork: picnic and ham	■ Pasteurized processed cheese spread and cheese food
■ Turkey: whole or drumsticks	
■ Chicken: whole, wings, or drumsticks	■ Some natural cheese, including brick, mozzarella, and cheddar
■ Dry peas	

$$ Thrifty Tips $$

$ Control meat portion size to control costs, as well as cholesterol and saturated fat. The correct serving size for meat is 2–3 oz. That's the size of the palm of a woman's hand or a deck of cards.

$ Make meat a side dish instead of the centerpiece of the meal. Smaller servings of meat mean bigger savings on your grocery bill.

$ Use less meat than is called for in a recipe. Often the amount can be reduced by 1/4 and not be missed. Use extra beans, rice, or pasta in soups, stews, and chili.

$ Try meatless meals several times a week. Use low-cost sources of protein, such as eggs, peanut butter, or dry beans. One egg, 1/4 cup of egg substitute, 2 egg whites, 2 tablespoons of peanut butter, or 1/2 cup of cooked dry beans is the protein equivalent of 1 oz of meat.

$ Don't use expensive cuts of meat in stews or casseroles.

$ Use less meat and more lettuce, tomatoes, and vegetables on sandwiches.

$ The least expensive cuts of meat are pork loin roast, boneless loin chops, boneless cooked ham, beef round, sirloin tip, and rump roast. Low fat content means less shrinkage and waste during cooking. These cuts should be covered during cooking and cooked a bit longer to tenderize.

$ Boneless cuts are often better buys, since you aren't paying for the weight of the bone. Think of cost per edible serving rather than cost per pound. Turkey has 46% edible meat per pound, while chicken has 41%.

$ Deli meat may be less expensive than prepackaged lunchmeats. Bake a small turkey breast or ham and slice it thinly for sandwiches.

$ Buy whole chickens on sale. Bone and skin the chicken yourself. Cut it and put it into individual packages of legs, breasts, and thighs to use as your recipes require. Drumsticks have a lower ratio of meat to bone and skin, so their edible portion costs are higher.

$ Wait for a sale, stock up, and then freeze boneless chicken breasts. You can get four servings per pound of chicken when you use it in stir-fry.

$ Make your own chicken tenders. Pound a boneless chicken breast to 1/2-inch thickness and cut it into strips using kitchen shears.

$ Tuna, salmon, and sardines canned in water, tomato sauce, or mustard are low-cost fish catches.

$ Ask for fish scraps at the fish counter in your grocery store. The scraps make wonderful chowders and soups.

$ Skip the store-made tuna or crab salad. It takes little time and money to make it yourself. Making it at home allows you to keep the fat content low.

$ Serve breakfast for dinner occasionally. A very economical omelet can be made with eggs, leftover vegetables, and cooked potatoes.

$ There is no nutritional difference between brown and white eggs. Choose white eggs since they cost less.

$ If there is less than a $0.07 difference between two sizes of the same grade of eggs, choose the larger egg for better value.

$ Why buy expensive egg substitutes? Two egg whites can replace one egg in a recipe. Two egg whites mixed with one whole egg can be substituted for two eggs.

$ Save money by buying a block of cheese and grating it yourself.

$ Use small amounts of strong-flavored cheeses, such as parmesan or sharp cheddar, rather than large amounts of milder cheeses. You'll save money and fat calories.

Fats, Sweets, and Alcohol

The foods at the tip of the pyramid should be eaten sparingly. Fats add flavor, but also calories. There is no suggested number of fat servings each day, but you should stay close to the number of grams or servings in your meal plan. Sweets are no longer off limits for people with diabetes. They can be eaten in small amounts, as long as they are substituted for other carbohydrates and as long as you know how they affect your blood glucose.

Alcohol has no nutrients and should be limited. The items in this section of the pyramid are mostly impulse purchases that are expensive for your health and your pocketbook. They add calories, but little or no nutrition for the money you spend.

$$ Thrifty Tips $$

$ Make your own cooking spray by putting vegetable oil in a spray bottle.

$ Olive oil is available in several grades. Use the costly extra virgin olive oil in dishes where its taste is apparent, such as salad dressings. Use a cheaper grade, such as virgin olive oil, in spicy dishes or dishes that will be heated.

$ Small bags of shelled walnuts, pecans, and almonds are costly. Buy a large bag on sale around the holidays and keep it in the freezer to use in cooking year-round. Buy loose nuts by the pound for even more savings.

$ Special diabetic or dietetic foods are no bargain. Case in point:

■ Fructose-sweetened peanut butter cup candy.
  Serving size: 5 pieces = 200 calories, 12 g fat, 19 g carbohydrate:
  Cost = $1.07

■ Sugar alcohol-sweetened peanut butter cup candy.
  Serving size: 5 pieces = 170 calories, 12 g fat, 24 g carbohydrate:
  Cost= $1.00

■ Regular peanut butter cup candy.
  Serving size: 5 pieces = 210 calories, 12 g fat, 22 g carbohydrate:
  Cost = $0.17

$ Rather than buying individual snack packs of pudding, make your own small servings from instant pudding mix and fat-free milk.

$ Two economical and healthy alternatives to sweet rolls and doughnuts are cinnamon toast made with your own homemade mix of cinnamon and sugar, and fruit spread or fruit butter on whole-wheat toast, English muffins, or bagels. Try "Apple-Prune Spread" on p. 129.

MISCELLANEOUS

There are various foods that don't fit anywhere into the pyramid; however, they can be big-cost items if purchased regularly. Luckily, there are cheap and effective ways of creating similar products for only a fraction of the cost. By being creative and using items you may already have around the house, you could save yourself a substantial amount of money.

$$ Thrifty Tips $$

Beverages

$ Sodas, carbonated fruit drinks, and flavored waters are poor choices for both nutritional and economical reasons. Use water as your main beverage and watch your food costs drop. Add a slice of lemon, lime, or orange for fruit taste and a twist of color.

$ Make your own combination juice drinks. It is cheaper to mix two juices together rather than purchase a premixed bottle of juice, such as cranberry-apple.

$ Beverages packed in sports bottles are premium priced.

$ Bottled tea, canned tea, or instant tea mix is far more expensive than tea made from tea bags. When purchasing tea, figure the cost based on the number of quarts you'll be able to make rather than on the weight of the jar or box.

$ Add a bit of ground cinnamon or a few drops of almond or vanilla extract to coffee grounds before brewing to make your own flavored coffee.

Herbs

$ Generic brands of herbs and spices can cost up to 50% less than brand names.

$ Buy small amounts of less frequently used dried herbs and spices.

$ Fresh herbs such as marjoram, oregano, rosemary, savory, and thyme freeze well.

$ Start your own herb garden. See Chapter 5.

Snacks

$ Pass on pricey low-fat cookies and chips. Low fat doesn't always mean healthy or low calorie.

$ Avoid individually packaged snacks. The cost of a single-serving bag of potato chips works out to over $5 per pound. Use carrot or celery sticks for crunch in lunch instead. Or try homemade chips, like the "Sassy Sweet Potato Chips" found on p. 91 for variety.

$ Penny-pinching healthy snacks include:

- Air-popped popcorn
- Unsalted pretzels
- Animal crackers
- Graham crackers
- Fresh fruit
- Raw vegetables
- Applesauce
- Unsweetened ready-to-eat cereal

100-CALORIE PORTIONS: DO IT YOURSELF

100-calorie portion packs of snack foods appeal to busy consumers who want to control portions, but would like someone else to do the math. Smart shoppers reap significant savings with a do-it-yourself approach. Consider carbohydrate content as well as calories for better blood glucose control.

Potato Crisps
100-calorie portion pack: $0.41 per tub
Do-It-Yourself version (9 potato crisps): $0.21

Fish Shaped Snack Crackers
100-calorie portion pack: $0.60 per packet
Do-It-Yourself version (39 crackers): $0.20

Teddy Bear Shaped Cookies
100-calorie portion pack: $0.48 per packet
Do-It-Yourself version (18 cookies): $0.24

Market Basket Makeover

Pyramid Penny-Pinching Saves Over 45%

Typical List	Smart Shopper List
Instant Oatmeal 12 packets = $3.69	Quick Cooking Oats 12 servings = $0.88
Lima Beans (frozen in butter) 10-oz package = $1.99	Lima Beans (frozen plain) 10-oz package = $0.89
Red Delicious Apples (loose) 5 lb = $6.45	Red Delicious Apples (bagged) 5 lb = $2.69
Liquid Egg Whites (1 egg white) = $0.19	Egg White (1 egg) = $0.10
Marinated Pork Tenderloin 1 lb = $6.39	Plain Pork Tenderloin 1 lb = $5.99
Brand Name Extra Virgin Olive Oil 17 oz = $8.49	Store Brand Extra Virgin Olive Oil 17 oz = $4.29
"Lite" Microwave Popcorn 1 serving = $0.35	Plain Popcorn (to air pop) 1 serving = $0.09
TOTAL $27.55	**TOTAL $14.93**

Money $aving Tip

Beans have been called the "poor man's meat" because they are an excellent alternative to meat, at only pennies per pound.

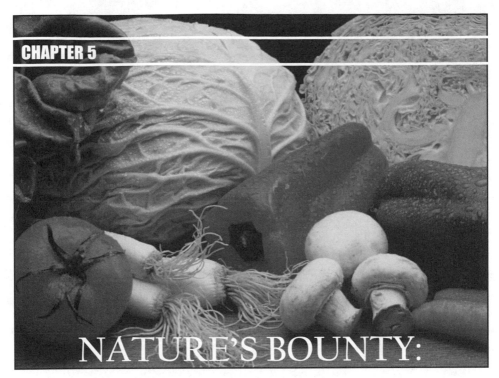

CHAPTER 5

NATURE'S BOUNTY:

HOW DOES YOUR GARDEN GROW?

G ardening is not a dirty word if you want to spend less and eat healthfully. In recent years, many people have stopped raising food in their own backyards because of lack of time or space. However, the bountiful benefits of gardening make it worth taking a second look.

Growing a garden is good for your wallet. For the price of a few starter plants or packets of seeds, you can enjoy fresh herbs or vegetables for months. Canning and freezing the fruits of your harvest ensures year-round savings. A stroll through your backyard garden, picking crisp green beans or juicy tomatoes for supper, or a look at your well-stocked pantry shelf and freezer, beats a trip to the produce aisle of your local store any time.

Gardening is work, but the physical activity it requires is an added benefit for people with diabetes, particularly those with type 2 diabetes who are trying to increase physical activity and reach a desirable body weight. The short list of sample gardening activities in the table that follows notes the calories burned per hour by a 150-pound person and lists the muscles used.

GARDENING ACTIVITY: SHAPING THE BODY		
Gardening Activity	**Calories Used**	**Muscles Used**
Planting seeds/plants	273 per hour	Arms, especially biceps and triceps
Pushing a wheelbarrow	341 per hour	Large muscle groups in the legs, especially quads and hamstrings
Pulling weeds	307 per hour	Full-body workout

Although gardening does require an investment of time, it can be a great stress-buster. The outdoor setting, physical activity, and sense of satisfaction from seeing the results of hard work bring peace of mind to many people who enjoy gardening as a hobby.

This chapter only peeks into the possibilities of gardening for fun and savings. Abundant resources are available through your local library, your state's Cooperative Extension Service office (under County Government in your telephone directory), and the Internet. Delve into gardening to create a dirt-cheap grocery bill!

HARVESTING HERBS

An herb garden is a wonderful place to begin perfecting your gardening skills. Herbs provide color, texture, and inviting aroma. They are versatile plants, used in a variety of ways from herb teas and jellies to flavored vinegars and oils for marinades, salad dressings, and sauces. Herbs are relatively easy to grow, whether on a sunny windowsill, in an outdoor container, or on a plot of backyard land.

INDOOR GARDENING

Windowsill herb gardening can be done with year-round favorites, such as oregano, chives, mint, rosemary, and thyme. Specific growing information for each herb variety is available where you buy your starter plants, but the following general guidelines will help you get growing.

Go for Sunshine

Select the sunniest window you have. Herbs require at least six hours of sunlight a day for the best development of their flavors. (Oregano is a particularly light-loving plant.) Your windowsill must be at least 5 inches wide to safely hold a 4-inch pot with a drainage saucer.

Start Small

Select small herb plants for starters, and transplant them into a premium-quality commercial potting mix in terra-cotta pots with plastic liners or rubber pads to catch leaks. Small containers require more frequent watering, especially since heated air indoors tends to dry plants out quickly.

Feed and Water

Check your plants every day, keeping the potting mix evenly moist by watering with a light spray. Remember that every watering leaches vital nutrients from the soil, so use a liquid feed to replace what has been washed away.

Leaves can be picked at any time of year, but for the best flavor, herbs should be harvested after their flower buds have formed and before they burst into bloom. Harvest your herbs in the morning when their oils are at their strongest. Cut only what you'll need to use for the day. Use sharp scissors to avoid bruising and to avoid loss of flavorful oils. Fresh herbs should enhance the flavor of food, not overwhelm it. Snip leaves with scissors, adding herbs to hot food at the last minute so they retain texture and color.

Cold dishes benefit from a sprinkling of herbs several hours before serving, or even overnight, to fully develop their flavor. A good rule of thumb is to use 1 tablespoon of fresh herbs to equal 1 teaspoon of crushed dried herbs in a recipe. Although herbs taste best when fresh from the garden, drying or freezing them will preserve any extras for future use.

THE GREAT OUTDOORS

If you have a bit more ambition and square footage, herbs can be grown outdoors in either a container or a garden plot. Container herb gardens, such as those grown in a half-barrel, are popular in cooler climates because they can be moved inside easily during cold snaps.

Herbs can become part of an existing vegetable garden or can be grown in their own small bed. A 4 × 6-foot space should easily accommodate a variety of herbs such as basil, cilantro, mint, oregano, parsley, rosemary, sage, tarragon, and thyme. The same tips for growing indoor herbs apply to those grown in containers or outdoor gardens, but there are special factors to take into consdieration when planting your garden outdoors.

Climate

Your local climate is the main influence on the variety of herbs you choose to grow. Most herbs will grow in all parts of the U.S., but the country is divided into 11 regions, or growing zones, dependent upon rainfall, sunshine, and temperature. Your state's Cooperative Extension Service will have complete information about your growing zone and which plants are most compatible with it.

Soil Quality

Soil quality is also key to the success of your garden. Some experts suggest that an herb garden bed be raised 10 or more inches off the ground for the best drainage. The soil should be a mixture of sterilized topsoil, peat moss, and sand or fine gravel. Testing the soil's pH is also a good idea; herbs thrive in a slightly acidic or near-neutral pH.

Location

Choose a sunny location for your garden and design it so that the perennial herbs (mint, oregano, rosemary, sage, tarragon, and thyme) are placed first. Then fill in the garden with annuals (such as basil and cilantro) and perhaps a biennial (parsley). Smaller herbs, such as oregano, parsley, and creeping thyme, belong in the front of the southern-facing exposure of your garden so that the taller plants like basil, tarragon, and cilantro, do not shade them. Allow plenty of space for herbs to grow so that they do not smother each other. In general, 18 inches between plants should be sufficient space.

Watering Plan

Finding the right watering plan for your outdoor herb garden may be a challenge. Herbs prefer dry soil, so they need only about an inch of water per week. Experienced gardeners use the soup can trick to measure the amount of water their plants are receiving. Place several soup cans among your herbs before you turn on your hose and note the time it takes to reach an inch of water in the cans. Use that as your guide for the proper watering time in the future. Water your herbs in the morning to give them time to dry out and to prevent fungus growth.

Just as good record keeping is important for your diabetes control, a diary of your herb-growing experiences is important for your herb garden's success. Note your successes and failures, complete with details on location, watering, and fertilizing, to ensure a better harvest from your garden in the future.

YOUR KITCHEN GARDEN

Raising food in the backyard was once a matter of survival. Most of us no longer live off the land, but homegrown produce does help to lower grocery costs. The best advice for a novice gardener is to start small and to think carefully about what you would like to plant. Your most valuable resource is your time. Spending hours toiling and tilling a plot of potatoes is not an economical use of your time if 10 pounds of potatoes are available at the grocery store for a minimal cost.

Plan ahead to grow the amount of produce you're able to consume, preserve, and store to avoid wasting time and resources. Your kitchen garden should be based on actual past grocery-store purchases of fruits and vegetables.

A productive vegetable garden of beans, beets, carrots, corn, cucumbers, lettuce, onions, peppers, tomatoes, and zucchini can be raised in a plot of land as small as 10 × 15 feet. The key elements of gardening—soil, water, sunlight, and seeds—remain the same no matter what the site. Your soil quality will be enhanced if you add organic matter, compost, and a balanced, natural fertilizer. Raised beds are recommended for easy reach and the most yield per square foot. Select a site close to your water source to save time and water. To receive maximum sun exposure, your garden should be set up so that the beds run from east to west.

The source of your garden plants is another place for savings. Fruits such as berries may be started from cuttings of existing plants. Most vegetables can be purchased in flats of seedlings from a nursery or garden center. Corn, carrots, beets, and beans are best started from seeds directly in the garden.

Bargains on vegetable seeds can be found if you catalog-shop or buy your seeds at season's end in a local store and hold them in a cool, dry place until the following year. Join a local garden club to tap into a wonderful source of advice, as well as perfectly good plants you get from other members at plant swaps and sales.

If a large garden plot is beyond the limits of your time and talents, a mini kitchen garden as small as 5 × 7 feet grown on a patio or balcony may be your solution. Lettuce, tomatoes, peppers, and eggplants adapt well to life in the concrete jungle if they are potted properly. Zucchini, snap beans, and cucumbers are other possibilities. Some varieties of cherry tomatoes can be grown in hanging baskets if they are carefully cared for. Put your windowsill to use and sprout pots of herbs or jars of seeds for future use.

FROM PLOT TO POT AND IN BETWEEN

Although the fruits of your garden taste best when freshly picked, it is also economical to store them for future use. There are a variety of storage methods available. The easiest and least expensive is the old-fashioned root cellar; carrots, potatoes, and onions do well there. However, many modern gardeners don't have the space for this method.

Dehydration

Fruits can be dehydrated into snacks. If you don't want to make the investment in a food dehydrator, sun drying, air drying, or drying in a low-temperature oven are other alternatives. Remember that dried fruits are concentrated sources of carbohydrates, and their serving size is usually quite small, approximately 1/4 cup.

Canning and Freezing

Home canning works for preserving almost everything in your garden, but it requires attention to many details, including pH levels, bacteria, processing time, and proper seals. Consult your county extension agent for information on the latest and safest canning methods.

Although a freezer is not a small investment, it can pay for itself over time with the money saved by preserving your harvest bounty. Some vegetables and fruits freeze better than others do. Vegetables freeze best if blanched (cooked in boiling water for a very short time) first so that they retain their color, flavor, and texture. Fruits can be packed and frozen in water, apple juice, or syrup. Reusable freezer containers are the least expensive way to store your harvest for future use.

Farmers' Markets

Finally, even if you don't have a green thumb, you can reap the money-saving benefits of gardening by looking for "pick your own" farms and farmers' markets in your area. According to the USDA, there are over 3,700 farmers markets operating in the United States. Take advantage of Mother Nature for penny-wise produce.

Money $aving Tip

Gardening is not only a great way to save money through growing your own fruits and vegetables, it's also a good source of physical activity.

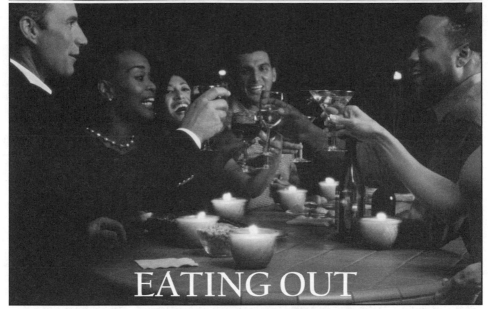

CHAPTER 6

EATING OUT
ON A LEAN BUDGET

I t's 4:00 in the afternoon. Maybe it has been a long day at work and you're tired. Maybe you're facing a busy evening of church, club, or children's activities. Maybe you've been under stress and want to treat yourself. These are the times when you are most likely to say, "I can't even think about cooking tonight." If you do, you certainly won't be alone.

On a typical day in the U.S., approximately 130 milion people are food service patrons. According to the USDA Economic Research Service Food Expenditure Chart, about $0.49 of every food dollar is spent on food prepared away from home, whether it be from a fast-food restaurant, home delivery, or takeout. Takeout foods are on the rise and projected to represent an even larger proportion of restaurant sales.

Does managing your diabetes meal plan on a budget mean an end to eating out? Of course not! As you can see from the meal plans in Chapter 2, it is possible to eat away from home and still spend less than $7 a day on food. You must learn to eat out economically, however, since it's likely you'll be eating away from home more frequently in the future. Industry experts predict a continued rise in restaurant dining. Careful planning on your part will prevent dining out from taking a big bite out of your budget.

Savings Strategies

Savings strategies for eating out can make a big dollar difference, especially if you consider that the average American spends close to $2,000 per year on food away from home. There are things you should keep in mind when you mull over your dining out options.

Face the Figures
Take a careful look at the amount of money you currently spend on food prepared away from home. Save your receipts, and track the amount you spend in a typical month. It may convince you to alter your eating habits. Dining away from home is an expensive convenience. Just one fast food value meal can be more expensive than an entire day's worth of healthy foods you prepare yourself.

Good Health Is Your Best Investment
It can be difficult to find nutritious and economical choices on the road. Invest in one of the many helpful books on the subject, such as the *Guide to Healthy Restaurant Eating, 3rd Edition*.

Plan Ahead
Try not to eat out impulsively. Think first about the planned-over meals you have ready at home. It may take just as much time to wait in a fast-food drive-through line as it would to microwave a much healthier pre-plated meal in your own kitchen. The savings are significant!

Make It Fast

It's said that the fastest growing appliance in America is not the microwave —it's the power window! Drivers today eat an average of 32 meals per year in their car. It's very likely you will drive through a fast food restaurant, grab a takeout meal, or order food to be delivered to your home sometime this week. In any given month, the average American consumes 24% of meals away from home. So what are some things you should keep in mind when eating on the run?

When Is a Value Meal Not a Value?

A value meal is no longer a value when it contains more food than you need to stick with your meal plan. If you want to order from the value menu, share your meal with a friend or family member. Consider selecting fruit, yogurt, or salad sides rather than fries for more nutrition and less fat.

Super Size Isn't Always Wise

You may be getting more food for the extra $0.67, but you are also buying about 400 extra calories on average, which may carry a price tag of its own in terms of weight gain and associated health care costs. If you must super size, share the meal with your dining companions.

Keep It Simple

Stick with foods in their simplest forms. A grilled chicken sandwich is generally cheaper and lower in fat and calories than the "deluxe" version. And eat like a child. The menu items marked "plain," "small," and "regular" are typically the best for your budget and your health.

Sub Shopping

Order a large version of your favorite healthy submarine sandwich and save half for another meal. The 12-inch size is often a better value than two 6-inch subs, and you'll benefit from the planned-overs tomorrow.

Chicken

When carrying out from a chicken restaurant or grocery store rotisserie display, order a whole chicken and several side items rather than individual boxed meals for your family. You will be better able to control portion sizes and extend the meal. Use leftover scraps for soups or casseroles.

Pizza Party

Always use coupons or ask for specials. Pizza makes great planned-overs for future meals. Refrigerate extra slices immediately to avoid overeating.

Beverage Bargains

Water is always your best bet as a beverage choice—and it's often free. Just ask for a cup of water rather than the pricey bottled waters. Fat-free milk and juices give you more nutrition bang for your buck than sodas or tea.

HAVE A SEAT

Surely it must have been a burned-out cook who said, "I'm making my favorite thing for dinner tonight—a reservation!" Getting out of the kitchen to enjoy a restaurant meal can be the highlight of the week. Use these pointers to enjoy your meal, yet stay within your food budget.

Choose a Restaurant for Taste—and Savings—Appeal

Eating in ethnic restaurants can be fun and inexpensive. For example, Chinese food is based on low-cost ingredients and cooking styles, so menu prices are reasonable. Food is often served family style, and sharing of dishes is encouraged—money saving strategies you'll love. Go meatless occasionally. Vegetarian restaurants offer healthful, low-cost options. Neighborhood restaurants may be less expensive than national chains.

Time Your Dining

Beat the clock by going to restaurants that offer early-bird specials. Also note that the very same menu items are often less expensive at lunch than at dinner. Portion sizes are more reasonable too. Breakfast items may be your best budget bet, no matter what time of day.

"Specials" Aren't Always Less Expensive

Listen carefully as the specials for the day are described, and don't be afraid to ask their prices. Although you may think the word "special" means money saving, it may be used to note the chef's specialty dish. There is no guarantee that it will be less expensive than the regular menu items.

Avoid Alcohol and Appetizers

Alcohol quickly adds up on your restaurant tab. Consider that you could buy a case of wine for what some restaurants charge for a bottle. Refrain from filling up on appetizers if you plan to order an entrée and side dishes.

Make Creative Meal Choices

Rather than feeling obliged to order an entrée for each person at the table, why not make more creative and inexpensive meal choices? For example, order a side salad for a starter and make an appetizer your main course. Also, eating family style by ordering a few entrées for the table and sharing them with your dining companions can result in cost savings.

Dessert Dilemma?

Often, there's the wish for "just a taste of something sweet" at the end of a meal. A good approach is to order a dessert to share with everyone. Try flavored decaffeinated coffee for another inexpensive sweet treat.

Is a Dining Card Program for You?

Discount dining cards or programs may save you up to 60% in participating restaurants. Investigate several options and keep in mind that there may be a fee for joining, as well as special requirements for obtaining discounts.

Consider a Coupon Book

Coupon books, containing coupons good toward food establishment purchases and services, are available for sale in most larger communities. There is often a minimal cost for purchase; however, using the coupons can quickly translate into several hundred dollars in savings each year.

Kids Eat Free

If you have children in tow, take advantage of "kids eat free" nights that many restaurants offer.

No matter which dining-out option you choose, remember:

A little knowledge goes a long way. You'll want to make smart nutrition choices, no matter which menu you're ordering from. Ask for nutrition information from the restaurants you eat at often. Many chains have pamphlets with the facts and figures you need. Or look for the nutrition information on their websites. Restaurants making nutrition claims for menu items, such as "light," "low fat", or "heart healthy", must comply with definitions established by the FDA and be able to provide nutrition information upon request.

Share and share alike. Restaurants are notorious for oversized portions. Take advantage of this by sharing with a dining companion. For example, one person would order a large salad and the other a traditional entrée.

Downsize. If you are without a dining companion to share oversized portions with and can't tote leftovers home, then ask for a half order or lunch-sized order to keep portions and cost in check.

Take it home. Another way to turn oversized restaurant portions to your advantage is to take home the leftovers. Ask for a "to go" container as your meal is being served, then pack up half right away so you won't be tempted to eat it all. You'll stay closer to the amount of food your body needs, as well as save money by already having tomorrow's lunch or dinner.

Money $aving Tip

When dining out, order several items from the menu and share them with your party. This will keeps costs and consumption lower than if you order and eat an entire entrée by yourself.

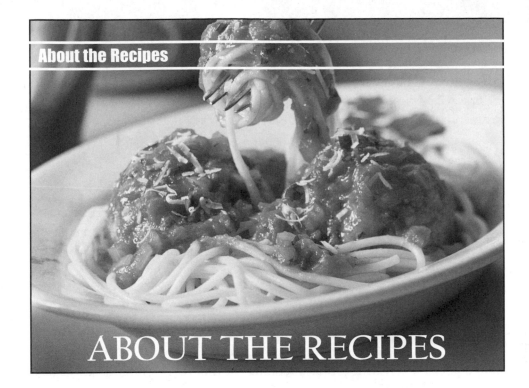

ABOUT THE RECIPES

The recipes in this book were carefully chosen to help you make the most of your precious resources: health, wealth, and time. They have passed the taste and convenience tests of busy families and professionals who want to eat healthfully without squandering their money or their minutes. Our recipes reflect the money-saving principles described in the pages of this book, including the concepts of planned-overs and batch cooking.

The preparation time is given for each recipe. This is the actual hands-on time it takes to prepare the ingredients for the recipe. Marinating time, chilling time, cooking time, etc. are also included. All of the recipes have been designed to improve your kitchen efficiency.

You may notice that the recipes are arranged a bit differently from the typical cookbook categories. They have been grouped according to their correct place on the Diabetes Food Pyramid from *The First Step in Diabetes Meal Planning.* You can easily refer back to Chapter 4 for helpful hints on choosing the most economical ingredients from each part of the food pyramid.

Notice that some of the recipes in one section can easily fit in a different section. For example, some dessert recipes from "Fats and Sweets" would be just as appropriate for "Fruits." This is another example of the versatility you can enjoy when planning your diabetes meals!

The recipes in this book were designed to meet the 2007 nutrition recommendations for people with diabetes.

Cost Analysis

The cost per serving and prices noted in the text and recipes were calculated based on local prices from a large national chain supermarket in summer 2007. These prices may vary based on the marketplace, the season of the year, and the area of the country.

Meat Prices
The prices on meat were the average sale prices (or the lowest price that could be found), since that's the recommended way to buy meat on a budget. Some of the meat prices required buying several pounds at once.

Produce Prices
Produce prices used were "in-season" prices.

Staple Ingredients
Prices for staple ingredients (flour, spices, broth, etc.) were for store brands when available and based on loyalty card or sale prices.

Packaged Items
Prices for cans, bottles, boxes, etc. based typically on the mid-range size—not the largest or smallest. Prices were for store brands when available and based on loyalty card or sale prices.

Optional Ingredients and Garnishes
Ingredients listed as optional or for garnish were not included in nutrient or cost analysis.

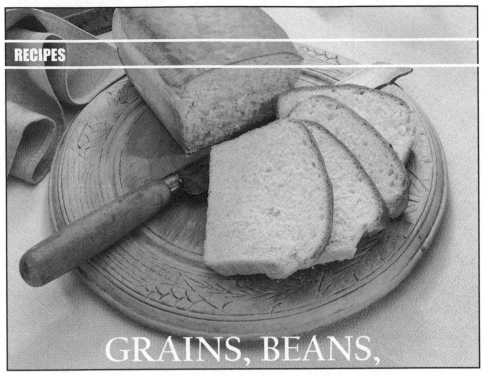

GRAINS, BEANS,

AND STARCHY VEGETABLES

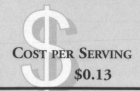

FIERY PINTO BEANS

PREPARATION TIME
20 minutes

COOKING TIME
2 1/2 hours

SERVINGS 26

SERVING SIZE 1/2 cup

EXCHANGES/ CHOICES
1 Starch

CALORIES 70
CALORIES FROM FAT 0

TOTAL FAT 0 g
SATURATED FAT <1 g
TRANS FAT 0 g

CHOLESTEROL 0 mg

SODIUM 160 mg

CARBOHYDRATE 12 g
DIETARY FIBER 4 g
SUGARS 1 g

PROTEIN 5 g

The cumin in this dish is used like a firefighter uses a hose—to cool down the heat! If you have any frozen leftover ham, just pull it out of the freezer for this recipe.

1 lb dried pinto beans
15 cups water, divided
1 cup chopped lean ham
1 large (approximately 8 oz) onion, chopped
1 4.5-oz can chopped green chilies
1 Tbsp ground cumin
1 Tbsp chili powder
1 tsp salt
1/4 tsp ground black pepper

1. Sort and wash beans, then place them in a 1-gallon stockpot. Add 10 cups of water, the ham, and the onion. Cover and bring to a boil over high heat.

2. Reduce heat until beans are at a simmer (a gentle boil), and simmer covered for 2 hours, stirring beans occasionally. Add remaining water, chilies, cumin, chili powder, salt, and pepper; then stir to combine.

3. Continue cooking an additional 30 minutes or unti beans are tender—again stirring periodically. If a thicker "soup" is desired, mash some of the beans with a spoon during this last half hour of cooking.

SIMPLE RED BEANS AND RICE

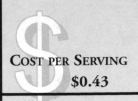

COST PER SERVING
$0.43

To remove the skin from fresh tomatoes, drop tomatoes in boiling water and leave them for 30 seconds. Remove with tongs and place gently in a pan of ice-cold water for 2 minutes. Tomato skins will easily peel off using your fingers.

Cooking spray
1 medium (approximately 5 oz) onion, chopped
1/2 medium (approximately 2–3 oz) green pepper, chopped
1 tsp minced garlic
1 Tbsp chili powder
1 tsp ground cumin
2 15.5-oz cans red beans, drained and rinsed
2 large (approximately 8 oz each) fresh tomatoes, peeled and chopped
1/2 cup mild picanté sauce
5 cups hot, cooked brown rice

1. Coat a large nonstick skillet with cooking spray anD warm over low-medium heat. Add onion, green pepper, and garlic and cook, stirring frequently, until onion is tender and translucent—about 5 minutes.

2. Add chili powder, cumin, beans, tomatoes, and picanté sauce. Cover and cook over low heat for 20 minutes.

3. Spoon 1/2 cup bean mixture over 1/2 cup rice to serve.

PREPARATION TIME
15 minutes

COOKING TIME
25 minutes

SERVINGS 10

SERVING SIZE
1/2 cup beans
1/2 cup rice

Exchanges/Choices
2 1/2 Starch
1 Vegetable

CALORIES 205
CALORIES FROM FAT 15

TOTAL FAT 2 g
SATURATED FAT <1 g
TRANS FAT 0 g

CHOLESTEROL 0 mg

SODIUM 215 mg

CARBOHYDRATE 41 g
DIETARY FIBER 7 g
SUGARS 4 g

PROTEIN 8 g

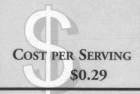

Sunday Afternoon Split Pea Soup

Preparation Time
15 minutes

Cooking Time
2 hours

Servings 8

Serving Size 1 cup

Exchanges/Choices
2 Starch
1 Lean Meat

Calories 215
Calories from Fat 20

Total Fat 2 g
Saturated Fat <1 g
Trans Fat 0 g

Cholesterol 15 mg

Sodium 345 mg

Carbohydrate 32 g
Dietary Fiber 12 g
Sugars 5 g

Protein 18 g

*A splendid soup to make on a lazy Sunday afternoon—
let the soup simmer on the stove while you rest on the
couch, then sit down to a filling meal of soup and Gran's
Country-Style Corn Bread (p. 80). Try this after the
holidays, using the holiday ham bone, boiling it with
the water and onion.*

12 cups water, divided
1 medium (approximately 5 oz) onion, finely diced
1 1/2 cups finely chopped lean ham
1 16-oz package dried split peas
2 tsp salt-free seasoning blend
1/8 tsp ground black pepper
Salt to taste (optional)

1. Place 10 cups water, onion, and ham in a 1-gallon
   stockpot over high heat and bring to a boil.

2. Meanwhile, place dried split peas in a colander and
   rinse under cool running water—remove any debris.
   Add peas to liquid and return to a boil.

3. Reduce heat until peas are at a simmer or a gentle boil,
   cover, and simmer for 1 1/2 hours, stirring periodically.
   Add remaining 2 cups water as needed during this
   cooking time.

4. Stir in salt-free seasoning blend and pepper and simmer
   over low heat for 15 minutes—soup should be thick.

Beth's Black-Eyed Peas

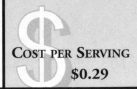
Serve as a side dish packed with fiber or over steaming rice for a filling main dish.

1 16-oz package dry black-eyed peas
8 cups cold water
6 cups warm water
2 cubes reduced-sodium beef bouillon
1 medium (approximately 5 oz) onion, finely diced
1/4 tsp salt

1. Rinse and sort peas. In a large pot, bring cold water and peas to a boil over high heat; boil for 2 minutes. Remove from heat, cover, and allow to soak for 1 hour. Drain off water and rinse peas.

2. Place soaked peas, warm water, bouillon cubes, and onion in a large pot. Bring to a boil over high heat. Reduce heat to low. Cook 45 minutes to 1 hour or until peas are tender, adding more warm water if necessary; stir periodically. Peas should be covered with a thick sauce.

3. Add salt, stir gently, and serve.

SOAKING TIME
1 hour

PREPARATION TIME
15 minutes

COOKING TIME
1 1/2 hours

SERVINGS 6

SERVING SIZE 1 cup

EXCHANGES/CHOICES
2 1/2 Starch
1 Lean Meat

CALORIES 235
CALORIES FROM FAT 10

TOTAL FAT 1 g
SATURATED FAT <1 g
TRANS FAT 0 g

CHOLESTEROL 0 mg

SODIUM 275 mg

CARBOHYDRATE 42 g
DIETARY FIBER 13 g
SUGARS 7 g

PROTEIN 15 g

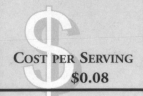

GRAN'S COUNTRY-STYLE CORN BREAD

PREPARATION TIME
5 minutes

BAKING TIME
20–25 minutes

SERVINGS 9

SERVING SIZE
1 square

EXCHANGES/CHOICES
1 1/2 Starch
1/2 Fat

CALORIES 140
CALORIES FROM FAT 20

TOTAL FAT 3 g
SATURATED FAT <1 g
TRANS FAT 0 g

CHOLESTEROL 25 mg

SODIUM 415 mg

CARBOHYDRATE 25 g
DIETARY FIBER 2 g
SUGARS 4 g

PROTEIN 5 g

For an extra special crunchy crust, try baking corn bread in a 9-inch iron skillet that has been heated in a 450°F oven and then coated generously with cooking spray. Turn bread out of pan as soon as it's baked.

1 3/4 cups self-rising white cornmeal mix
1/4 cup all-purpose flour
1 egg
2 tsp corn oil
1 1/2 cups low-fat buttermilk

1. Preheat oven to 450°F. Place all ingredients in large mixing bowl and stir to combine.

2. Pour into 9 × 9-inch baking pan coated generously with cooking spray, and bake for 20 to 25 minutes or until corn bread is golden brown.

3. Slice into 3 × 3-inch squares.

QUICK GARLIC BUNS

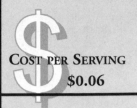

COST PER SERVING
$0.06

Here's an imaginative and yummy way to use extra hamburger or hot dog buns, even if they are slightly stale.

3 hamburger or hot dog buns
6 tsp light tub margarine
1/4 tsp garlic salt

1. Preheat broiler. Open buns and lay on a baking sheet with the crust side down.

2. In a small bowl, combine margarine and garlic salt. Spread each bun half with 1 tsp of the margarine and garlic salt mixture.

3. Place in oven 5 inches from broiler, and broil with door slightly cracked until margarine is melted and buns are lightly toasted, about 3 minutes.

PREPARATION TIME
5 minutes

BROILING TIME
3 minutes

SERVINGS 6

SERVING SIZE 1/2 bun

EXCHANGES/CHOICES
1 Starch

CALORIES 75
CALORIES FROM FAT 20

TOTAL FAT 3 g
SATURATED FAT <1 g
TRANS FAT 0 g

CHOLESTEROL 0 mg

SODIUM 185 mg

CARBOHYDRATE 11 g
DIETARY FIBER 0 g
SUGARS 1 g

PROTEIN 2 g

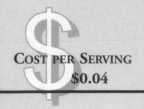

COST PER SERVING
$0.04

CRUNCHY CROUTONS

PREPARATION TIME
10 minutes

BAKING TIME
9 minutes

SERVINGS 4

SERVING SIZE
16 croutons

EXCHANGES/CHOICES
1 Starch
1/2 Fat

CALORIES 90
CALORIES FROM FAT 30

TOTAL FAT 4 g
SATURATED FAT <1 g
TRANS FAT 0 g

CHOLESTEROL 0 mg

SODIUM 260 mg

CARBOHYDRATE 12 g
DIETARY FIBER 1 g
SUGARS 1 g

PROTEIN 2 g

Here's an economical way to use stale bread! These are tasty sprinkled on a green salad or a steaming bowl of soup.

1/2 tsp garlic salt
1/8 tsp onion powder
2 Tbsp light tub margarine, melted
4 slices white bread

1. Preheat oven to 400°F.

2. Stir garlic salt and onion powder into melted margarine. Using a pastry brush, coat both sides of each slice of bread with the margarine mixture, then lay bread on baking sheet. Cut bread into 1-inch cubes (16 per slice) and separate the cubes on the baking sheet.

3. Bake for 5 minutes, stir, then continue to bake until golden and crispy, about 4 minutes.

BANANA-OATMEAL MUFFINS

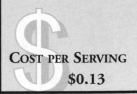

COST PER SERVING
$0.13

If you're making these muffins for breakfast, combine the dry ingredients the night before to save time in the morning.

1 cup old-fashioned rolled oats
3/4 cup fat-free milk
1 cup all-purpose flour
1/3 cup sugar
1 Tbsp baking powder
1/4 tsp salt
1/4 tsp cinnamon
1 egg, well beaten
3 Tbsp corn oil
1 medium (approximately 6 oz) ripe banana, mashed
Cooking spray

1. Preheat oven to 425°F. In a large mixing bowl, stir together oats and milk, then let stand 15 minutes.

2. In a separate bowl, sift together flour, sugar, baking powder, salt, and cinnamon. In a third bowl, combine egg, oil, and banana.

3. Add banana mixture to oat mixture. Stir in dry ingredients.

4. Line muffin pan with 12 paper baking cups, and coat with cooking spray. Spoon batter into baking cups, filling 3/4 full. Bake for 15 minutes or until muffins are golden and spring back when touched. Cool on rack.

PREPARATION TIME
25 minutes

BAKING TIME
15 minutes

SERVINGS 12

SERVING SIZE
1 muffin

EXCHANGES/CHOICES
1 1/2 Carbohydrate
1/2 Fat

CALORIES 135
CALORIES FROM FAT 40

TOTAL FAT 5 g
SATURATED FAT <1 g
TRANS FAT 0 g

CHOLESTEROL 20 mg

SODIUM 155 mg

CARBOHYDRATE 22 g
DIETARY FIBER 1 g
SUGARS 8 g

PROTEIN 3 g

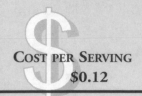

GOLDEN APPLESAUCE MUFFINS

PREPARATION TIME
15 minutes

BAKING TIME
16–20 minutes

SERVINGS 12

SERVING SIZE
1 muffin

EXCHANGES/ CHOICES
1 1/2 Carbohydrate

CALORIES 115
CALORIES FROM FAT 5

TOTAL FAT 1 g
SATURATED FAT <1 g
TRANS FAT 0 g

CHOLESTEROL 20 mg

SODIUM 185 mg

CARBOHYDRATE 24 g
DIETARY FIBER 2 g
SUGARS 9 g

PROTEIN 4 g

Applesauce lends a sweet flavor and replaces oil in these moist muffins.

1 1/4 cups all-purpose flour
1/2 tsp baking powder
1/2 tsp baking soda
1/8 tsp salt
1/3 cup sugar
2 cups bran flake cereal, crushed
1 1/4 cups fat-free milk
1 egg, beaten
1/3 cup unsweetened applesauce
Cooking spray

1. Preheat oven to 400°F. In a mixing bowl, combine flour, baking powder, baking soda, salt, and sugar.

2. In a separate large mixing bowl, combine bran flakes and milk, then let stand until cereal is softened, about 2 minutes.

3. Stir in egg and applesauce, mixing well. Add dry ingredients and stir just until combined.

4. Line muffin tin with 12 paper baking cups, and coat with cooking spray. Spoon batter into baking cups, filling 3/4 full. Bake for 16–20 minutes, until muffins are golden and spring back when touched. Cool on rack.

CINNAMON FRENCH TOAST

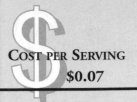

COST PER SERVING
$0.07

This is a super way to use day-old or slightly stale bread. Try it with Wild Berry Syrup (p. 189).

1 egg + 2 egg whites
1/2 cup fat-free milk
1/4 tsp vanilla extract
1/8 tsp cinnamon
8 slices bread
Butter-flavored cooking spray

1. In a shallow dish, whisk together egg and egg whites, milk, vanilla, and cinnamon. Dip each slice of bread quickly in egg mixture to coat one side, flip over with fork, and quickly coat other side.

2. Place in large nonstick skillet coated generously with cooking spray and warmed over medium heat. Cook until golden, turn over, and continue cooking until other side is golden. If cooking French toast in 2 batches, recoat skillet with cooking spray between batches.

PREPARATION TIME
5 minutes

BAKING TIME
8–10 minutes

SERVINGS 8

SERVING SIZE
1 slice

EXCHANGES/CHOICES
1 Starch

CALORIES 80
CALORIES FROM FAT 15

TOTAL FAT 2 g
SATURATED FAT <1 g
TRANS FAT 0 g

CHOLESTEROL 25 mg

SODIUM 155 mg

CARBOHYDRATE 13 g
DIETARY FIBER 1 g
SUGARS 1 g

PROTEIN 4 g

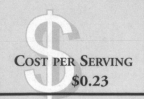

SPICED RAISIN BREAD PUDDING

PREPARATION TIME
25 minutes

BAKING TIME
30 minutes

SERVINGS 10

SERVING SIZE
1/2 cup

EXCHANGES/CHOICES
2 Carbohydrate
1 Fat

CALORIES 175
CALORIES FROM FAT 45

TOTAL FAT 5 g
SATURATED FAT 1 g
TRANS FAT 0 g

CHOLESTEROL 20 mg

SODIUM 280 mg

CARBOHYDRATE 26 g
DIETARY FIBER 1 g
SUGARS 13 g

PROTEIN 5 g

This is a simple way to transform day-old bread into a marvelous dessert. If the bread is not very dry, bake it in the oven at 350°F for 5 minutes to dry it out.

2 cups fat-free milk
4 Tbsp light tub margarine
6 cups cubed, dry day-old French bread
1 egg + 2 egg whites
1/2 tsp ground cloves
1 1/2 tsp cinnamon
1/4 tsp salt
1 tsp vanilla extract
3 Tbsp packed Splenda brown sugar blend
2 Tbsp Splenda sugar blend for baking
1/2 cup raisins
Cooking spray

1. Preheat oven to 350°F. Warm milk and margarine in a very large (5 quart) saucepan over medium heat until margarine is melted—do not boil. Remove from heat, stir in bread, and cool 10 minutes.

2. Meanwhile, combine egg and egg whites in a bowl and whisk until foamy. Mix in cloves, cinnamon, salt, vanilla extract, brown sugar, and baking mix. Add to cooled milk/bread and stir to combine.

3. Mix in raisins, and spoon pudding into 2-quart casserole dish coated with cooking spray. Bake for 30 minutes or until pudding is set and a toothpick inserted into the center of the pudding comes out clean.

TEMPTING TOMATO AND MACARONI MEDLEY

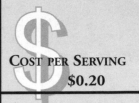

COST PER SERVING
$0.20

If fresh tomatoes are not in season, you can substitute 2 14.5-oz cans diced tomatoes, drained.

1 3/4 cups uncooked elbow macaroni
4 cups peeled, diced tomatoes
1 Tbsp + 1 tsp corn oil
1/4 tsp ground black pepper
1/8 tsp salt
1/8 tsp garlic powder

1. In a large pan, cook macaroni according to package directions, omitting salt if called for. Drain macaroni, return to pan, and add remaining ingredients.

2. Simmer uncovered over medium-low heat for 20 minutes or until tomatoes have cooked down—stir gently to prevent sticking.

PREPARATION TIME
10 minutes

BAKING TIME
30 minutes

SERVINGS 14

SERVING SIZE
1/2 cup

EXCHANGES/CHOICES
1 Starch

CALORIES 85
CALORIES FROM FAT 20

TOTAL FAT 2 g
SATURATED FAT <1 g
TRANS FAT 0 g

CHOLESTEROL 0 mg

SODIUM 25 mg

CARBOHYDRATE 15 g
DIETARY FIBER 1 g
SUGARS 1 g

PROTEIN 3 g

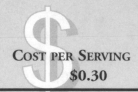

COST PER SERVING
$0.30

CHEESY CORN ON THE COB

PREPARATION TIME
10 minutes

COOKING TIME
15 minutes

STANDING TIME
5 minutes

SERVINGS 8

SERVING SIZE
1 ear

EXCHANGES/ CHOICES
1 1/2 Starch
1/2 Fat

CALORIES 130
CALORIES FROM FAT 35

TOTAL FAT 4 g
SATURATED FAT 1 g
TRANS FAT 0 g

CHOLESTEROL 0 mg

SODIUM 215 mg

CARBOHYDRATE 21 g
DIETARY FIBER 3 g
SUGARS 3 g

PROTEIN 5 g

One bite and you'll fall in love with corn.

8 medium (approximately 5 oz each) ears of corn, husks
　　and silks removed
3 Tbsp light tub margarine, melted
1/4 tsp garlic salt
4 slices fat-free American cheese

1. Fill a 1-gallon pot half full with water and bring to a
　　boil over high heat. Add corn and boil for 7 minutes
　　or until kernels are tender. Drain corn.

2. In a small bowl, combine melted margarine and garlic
　　salt. Using a pastry brush, coat corn with margarine
　　mixture.

3. Place in serving dish and lay 1/2 slice of cheese over
　　each ear of corn. Allow to stand for 5 minutes before
　　serving so that cheese melts.

RICE ROYALE

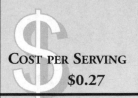
To make canned beef bouillon less fattening, chill bouillon in the refrigerator for at least 1 hour, then skim off the fat that rises to the top.

3 Tbsp light tub margarine
1 cup uncooked brown rice
1 7-oz can mushroom stems and pieces, drained
1/2 cup finely chopped onion
1 14.5-oz can fat-free, 50% reduced-sodium beef
   broth
1/8 tsp ground black pepper
1 Tbsp chopped fresh parsley

1. Melt margarine in a large nonstick skillet over medium-high heat. Add uncooked rice, mushrooms, and onion. Cook, stirring constantly, until rice is golden (about 5 minutes).

2. Stir in beef broth and black pepper. Bring to a boil. Reduce heat to low, cover, and cook until rice is tender and liquid is absorbed (about 15 to 20 minutes)—stir periodically.

3. Fluff rice with a fork, sprinkle with parsley, and serve.

PREPARATION TIME
5 minutes

COOKING TIME
30 minutes

SERVINGS 8

SERVING SIZE
1/2 cup

EXCHANGES/CHOICES
1 Starch
1 Vegetable
1 Fat

CALORIES 140
CALORIES FROM FAT 40

TOTAL FAT 5 g
SATURATED FAT 1 g
TRANS FAT 0 g

CHOLESTEROL 0 mg

SODIUM 205 mg

CARBOHYDRATE 21 g
DIETARY FIBER 3 g
SUGARS 1 g

PROTEIN 4 g

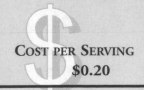

OVEN-BAKED SWEET POTATOES WITH MAPLE CREAM

PREPARATION TIME
10 minutes

COOKING TIME
45–60 minutes

SERVINGS 8

SERVING SIZE
1/2 potato
1/2 Tbsp cream

EXCHANGES/CHOICES
1 Starch

CALORIES 65
CALORIES FROM FAT 0

TOTAL FAT 0 g
SATURATED FAT 0 g
TRANS FAT 0 g

CHOLESTEROL 0 mg

SODIUM 25 mg

CARBOHYDRATE 14 g
DIETARY FIBER 2 g
SUGARS 5 g

PROTEIN 2 g

To save time, try microwaving the potatoes rather than oven baking them. The maple cream is also tasty drizzled over cut up fresh fruit.

4 medium (approximately 5 oz each) sweet potatoes
1/4 cup fat-free sour cream
1 Tbsp maple syrup
1/8 tsp vanilla extract
1/4 tsp cinnamon

1. Preheat oven to 400°F. Wash and dry potatoes. Pierce each 5 times with a fork and place on a baking sheet. Bake at 400°F for 45–60 minutes or until tender when pierced with a fork.

2. In a small bowl, whisk together sour cream, syrup, and vanilla extract.

3. Split each potato lengthwise, taking care not to cut all the way through. Spoon 1/2 Tbsp maple cream over each half of a split potato, and sprinkle with cinnamon.

Sassy Sweet Potato Chips

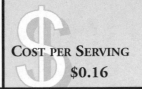

Cost per Serving
$0.16

Chili powder and cumin complement the sweetness of these chips.

4 medium (approximately 5 oz each) sweet potatoes
4 tsp corn oil
1/4 tsp chili powder
1/4 tsp ground cumin
1/8 tsp ground black pepper
1/4 tsp salt
Cooking spray

1. Preheat oven to 375°F. Peel sweet potatoes, slice into 1/8-inch-thick slices, then place in a bowl or baking pan.

2. Combine oil and seasonings in a small bowl. Drizzle over potatoes, then toss to coat potato slices well.

3. Place potato slices in a single layer on a baking pan coated with cooking spray. Bake for 10 minutes. Turn chips over and bake an additional 30 minutes, turning chips every 10 minutes. To prevent heat loss, remove pan from oven and close oven door when turning chips. (Watch closely during last 5 minutes of baking to prevent burning—you may need to remove smaller chips early.)

4. Transfer chips to wire rack to cool.

Preparation Time
20 minutes

Cooking Time
40 minutes

Servings 10

Serving Size
1/2 cup

Exchanges/Choices
1/2 Starch
1/2 Fat

Calories 50
Calories from Fat 20

Total Fat 2 g
Saturated Fat <1 g
Trans Fat 0 g

Cholesterol 0 mg

Sodium 70 mg

Carbohydrate 8 g
Dietary Fiber 1 g
Sugars 3 g

Protein 1 g

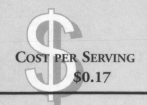

Seasoned Potato Skin Crisps

Preparation Time
15 minutes

Baking Time
1 hour, 40 minutes

Cooking Time
10 minutes

Servings 6

Serving Size
1 whole potato skin

Exchanges/Choices
2 Starch
1/2 Fat

Calories 150
Calories from Fat 35

Total Fat 4 g
Saturated Fat <1 g
Trans Fat <1 g

Cholesterol 0 mg

Sodium 120 mg

Carbohydrate 27 g
Dietary Fiber 5 g
Sugars 1 g

Protein 3 g

Stir chopped chives into fat-free sour cream for a terrific topper!

6 medium (approximately 5 oz each) baking potatoes
2 1/2 Tbsp light stick margarine
1/4 tsp seasoned salt
1/8 tsp garlic powder
Paprika

1. Preheat oven to 400°F. Wrap clean potatoes in foil and bake for 1 hour and 15 minutes or until tender when pierced with a fork. Unwrap potatoes, cut in half lengthwise, and cool 10 minutes to prevent a burn and allow easier slicing.

2. Scoop out potato pulp (a melon-ball scoop works well), leaving a 1/4-inch layer of pulp on skin. Set pulp aside (can use to make mashed potatoes). Gently cut potato skins lengthwise into 1-inch strips (4–6 strips per potato).

3. In a small saucepan, melt margarine. Stir in seasoned salt and garlic powder. Using a pastry brush, coat potato skins with seasoned margarine.

4. Place skins on two baking sheets and bake for 25 minutes or until crisp. Sprinkle with paprika before serving.

Roasted Barbecue Potatoes

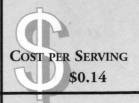
COST PER SERVING
$0.14

These potatoes make a nice complement to sizzling hamburgers just off the grill.

6 medium (approximately 5 oz each) baking potatoes, unpeeled
Cooking spray
1 large (approximately 8 oz) onion, thinly sliced and separated into rings
3 Tbsp all-purpose flour
2 1/4 cups cold water
3/4 cup barbecue sauce
1 Tbsp white vinegar
1/4 tsp salt
1/8 tsp ground black pepper

1. Preheat oven to 375°F. Thinly slice (1/8 inch thick) potatoes and layer in a 9 × 13-inch pan coated with cooking spray. Top potatoes with onion rings and set aside.

2. In a large bowl, whisk together flour and water. Whisk in barbecue sauce, vinegar, salt, and pepper. Pour over potatoes, cover with foil, and bake for 1 hour—stir every 30 minutes.

3. Remove foil after 1 hour baking time, return potatoes to oven, and continue baking an additional 45 minutes or until potatoes are tender when pierced with a fork.

PREPARATION TIME
15 minutes

BAKING TIME
1 hour, 45 minutes

SERVINGS 12

SERVING SIZE
1/2 potato, or
1/12 recipe

EXCHANGES/CHOICES
1 1/2 Carbohydrate

CALORIES 90
CALORIES FROM FAT 0

TOTAL FAT 1 g
SATURATED FAT <1 g
TRANS FAT <1 g

CHOLESTEROL 0 mg

SODIUM 90 mg

CARBOHYDRATE 15 g
DIETARY FIBER 1 g
SUGARS 1 g

PROTEIN 1 g

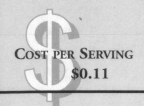

COST PER SERVING
$0.11

SKILLET POTATOES

This versatile dish is a country-style favorite. Serve it up in your most colorful bowl as a side for almost any breakfast, lunch, or supper!

4 medium (approximately 5 oz each) potatoes, unpeeled, thinly sliced
Cooking spray
1 small (approximately 3 oz) onion, sliced and separated into rings
1 1/2 cups water
1 Tbsp light margarine
1/4 tsp salt
1/8 tsp ground black pepper
1/4 tsp garlic powder

1. Spread potatoes over bottom of a large nonstick skillet coated with cooking spray. Cover with rings of onion. Pour water over potatoes and onions, then dot with margarine. Cover skillet and cook over medium-high heat for 15 minutes or until potatoes are tender.

2. Remove lid and continue cooking, allowing liquid to evaporate—do not stir. Sprinkle potatoes and onions evenly with salt, pepper, and garlic powder.

3. When potatoes dry, turn them over gently with a spatula (some slices may break). Continue cooking an additional 5 minutes. Potatoes will be tender with some slices a light golden brown.

Carrots, Onions, and Potatoes

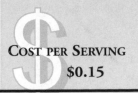

This vegetable medley makes a savory accompaniment to the Dijon-Crusted Beef Roast, p. 160—both recipes bake at the same temperature.

3 carrots (approximately 3 oz each), peeled and sliced into
   1/2-inch chunks
1 large (approximately 8 oz) onion, sliced and separated
   into rings
1 1/2 large potatoes, peeled and cut into bite-sized
   chunks (approximately 1 1/2 lbs)
1 Tbsp light margarine
1/4 tsp salt
1/4 tsp ground black pepper
1/8 tsp garlic powder
1/2 cup fat-free, 50% reduced-sodium chicken broth

1. Preheat oven to 325°F. Place carrots, onion, potatoes, and margarine on a large piece of wide foil, and then place foil with vegetables in a 9 × 13-inch baking pan.

2. Sprinkle vegetables evenly with salt, pepper, and garlic powder. Drizzle chicken broth over top. Seal foil to make a packet. Bake for 1 1/2 hours or until vegetables are tender.

3. Use caution when opening the packet to avoid being burned by hot steam! Stir vegetables to coat, then serve.

Preparation Time
15 minutes

Baking Time
1 1/2 hours

Servings 12

Serving Size
1/2 cup

Exchanges/ Choices
1/2 Starch
1 Vegetable

Calories 60
Calories from Fat 10

Total Fat 1 g
Saturated Fat <1 g
Trans Fat <1 g

Cholesterol 0 mg

Sodium 95 mg

Carbohydrate 12 g
Dietary Fiber 2 g
Sugars 2 g

Protein 1 g

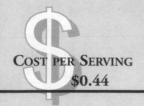

COST PER SERVING
$0.44

CREAMY PEAS WITH MUSHROOMS

PREPARATION TIME
5 minutes

COOKING TIME
15 minutes

SERVINGS 4

SERVING SIZE
1/2 cup

EXCHANGES/CHOICES
1 Starch
1 Fat

CALORIES 130
CALORIES FROM FAT 45

TOTAL FAT 5 g
SATURATED FAT 1 g
TRANS FAT < 1 g

CHOLESTEROL 0 mg

SODIUM 390 mg

CARBOHYDRATE 16 g
DIETARY FIBER 3 g
SUGARS 6 g

PROTEIN 6 g

Here's another complementary side dish for Dijon-Crusted Beef Roast, p. 160.

2 Tbsp light tub margarine
1/2 medium (approximately 3 oz) onion, chopped
1 Tbsp all-purpose flour
1/4 tsp salt
Dash ground black pepper
1 cup fat-free milk
1 cup sliced fresh mushrooms
1 14.5-oz can peas, drained and rinsed

1. In a nonstick skillet, melt margarine over medium heat. Add onion and sauté until tender. Stir in flour, salt, and pepper—will be pasty.

2. Add milk and mix with a wire whisk until thickened and bubbly, about 3 minutes. Add mushrooms, then cook and stir for 2 minutes.

3. Reduce heat to medium-low, add peas, and cook 5 additional minutes, stirring periodically.

SAVORY POTATO SOUP

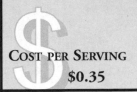
*It's the perfect warm-up on a chilly winter's evening—
and it's great reheated for lunch too!*

5 cups peeled and cubed potatoes (approximately 2 lbs)
3 cups fat-free milk
1 cup water
3 cubes reduced-sodium chicken bouillon
2 medium (approximately 5 oz each) onions, finely
    chopped
1/2 cup (approximately 1 medium rib) celery, finely
    chopped
1 Tbsp light margarine
3/4 tsp salt
1/4 tsp ground black pepper
1/8 tsp garlic powder

1. Place potatoes in a large Dutch oven, cover with water,
   and cook over medium-high heat until potatoes are
   tender when pierced with a fork (about 15 minutes).
   Drain off water.

2. Remove approximately half of potatoes, mash with a
   potato masher, then return to pan.

3. Add milk, 1 cup water, bouillon, onion, celery,
   margarine, salt, pepper, and garlic powder to potatoes.
   Simmer uncovered for 30 minutes or until mixture
   thickened and is heated through. Stir periodically to
   prevent sticking.

PREPARATION TIME
25 minutes

COOKING TIME
1 hour

SERVINGS 7

SERVING SIZE
1 cup

EXCHANGES/CHOICES
1 1/2 Starch
1/2 Milk
1 Vegetable

CALORIES 170
CALORIES FROM FAT 15

TOTAL FAT 2 g
SATURATED FAT <1 g
TRANS FAT <1 g

CHOLESTEROL 0 mg

SODIUM 550 mg

CARBOHYDRATE 33 g
DIETARY FIBER 3 g
SUGARS 9 g

PROTEIN 6 g

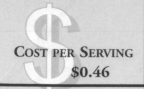

Cost per Serving
$0.46

Rainbow Dill and Cucumber Pasta Salad

Fresh from the garden vegetables and colorful pasta make this a fun recipe for a potluck!

PREPARATION TIME
20 minutes

COOKING TIME
10–12 minutes

SERVINGS 8

SERVING SIZE
1 cup

EXCHANGES/CHOICES
2 Starch
1 Vegetable
1/2 Fat

CALORIES 194
CALORIES FROM FAT 29

TOTAL FAT 3 g
SATURATED FAT 2 g
TRANS FAT 0 g

CHOLESTEROL 12 mg

SODIUM 111 mg

CARBOHYDRATE 33 g
DIETARY FIBER 2 g
SUGARS 5 g

PROTEIN 8 g

Pasta
4 cups rainbow twirl pasta

Dressing
1 cup reduced-fat sour cream
1/2 cup fat-free milk
1 Tbsp chopped fresh dill weed
1 tsp coarse ground black pepper
1/4 tsp salt
1 Tbsp distilled white vinegar
1 medium (approximately 5 oz) cucumber, peeled, seeded, and chopped
1 medium (approximately 5 oz) tomato, chopped
1/2 cup chopped red onion
1 cup broccoli florets

1. Cook pasta according to package directions, without additional oil or salt. Drain and rinse in cold water. Transfer noodles to a large bowl.

2. In a separate bowl, mix together sour cream, milk, dill, pepper, salt, and vinegar. Set dressing aside.

3. Mix cucumber, tomato, onion, and broccoli into the pasta. Pour in dressing and mix thoroughly. Cover and refrigerate at least 1 hours and preferably overnight. Stir just before serving.

BUTTERNUT SQUASH SOUP

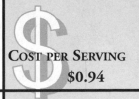
COST PER SERVING
$0.94

A fall favorite!

1 small (approximately 3 oz) onion, finely chopped
4 Tbsp light margarine
6 cups peeled and cubed butternut squash (approximately
  2 lbs)
3 cups water
4 cubes reduced-sodium chicken bouillon
1/2 tsp dried marjoram
1/4 tsp ground black pepper
1/4 tsp ground cayenne pepper
2 8-oz packages fat-free cream cheese

1. In a large saucepan, sauté onions in margarine until
   tender. Add squash, water, bouillon, marjoram, and
   peppers. Bring to boil; cook 20 minutes or until squash
   is tender.

2. Puree squash and cream cheese in a blender or food
   processor in batches until smooth. Return to saucepan
   and heat through. Do not allow to boil.

PREPARATION TIME
25 minutes

COOKING TIME
35 minutes

SERVINGS 6

SERVING SIZE
  1 cup

EXCHANGES
  1 Lean Meat
  1 Fat

CALORIES 166
CALORIES FROM FAT 32

TOTAL FAT 4 g
SATURATED FAT 1 g
TRANS FAT 0 g

CHOLESTEROL 9 mg

SODIUM 942 mg

CARBOHYDRATE 19 g
DIETARY FIBER 1 g
SUGARS 6 g

PROTEIN 12 g

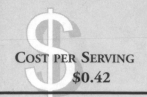

CONFETTI WILD RICE SALAD

A quick, colorful, and delicious way to use leftover rice.

PREPARATION TIME
15 minutes

CHILLING TIME
1 hour

SERVINGS 11

SERVING SIZE
1/2 cup

EXCHANGES/ CHOICES
1 Starch
1 Fat

CALORIES 135
CALORIES FROM FAT 57

TOTAL FAT 6 g
SATURATED FAT 1 g
TRANS FAT 0 g

CHOLESTEROL 2 mg

SODIUM 343 mg

CARBOHYDRATE 17 g
DIETARY FIBER 1 g
SUGARS 1 g

PROTEIN 3 g

Salad
2 oz crumbled reduced-fat feta cheese
1/2 cup finely chopped green bell pepper
1/2 cup finely chopped red onion
1/2 cup finely chopped tomato
2 oz black olives, chopped
4 cups cooked long grain and wild rice

Dressing
1/4 cup olive oil
3 Tbsp red wine vinegar
1/2 tsp dried tarragon
1/8 tsp black pepper

1. In a large bowl, combine feta, green pepper, onion, tomato, olives, and rice; stir to mix well.

2. In a small bowl, whisk together olive oil, vinegar, tarragon, and pepper.

3. Pour dressing over salad and stir to coat well.

4. Cover and refrigerate for at least 1 hour to allow flavors to blend.

HEARTY OATMEAL FOR ONE

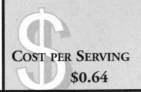

Double the recipe to share with a friend or enjoy the next day. Reheat and thin with milk or water. Add banana, yogurt, and honey right before serving.

1 cup fat-free milk
1/2 cup quick oats
1 Tbsp maple syrup
1 Tbsp raisins
2 dashes cinnamon
2 dashes nutmeg
1 Tbsp flaked coconut
1 Tbsp chopped walnuts
1/4 medium (approximately 1 1/2 oz) banana, sliced
2 Tbsp no sugar added, fat-free vanilla yogurt
1 tsp honey

1. Pour the milk into a saucepan and bring to a simmer over medium-high heat.

2. Stir in the oats, syrup, raisins, cinnamon, and nutmeg. Return to a simmer, then reduce heat to medium and cook for 1–2 minutes.

3. Stir in coconut and walnuts and let stand until oatmeal reaches desired thickness.

4. Top with banana and yogurt, then drizzle with honey.

PREPARATION TIME
10 minutes

SERVINGS 1

SERVING SIZE
1 1/2 cups

EXCHANGES/CHOICES
2 Starch
1 Fat
1 Fruit
1 Milk

CALORIES 460
CALORIES FROM FAT 84

TOTAL FAT 9 g
SATURATED FAT 3 g
TRANS FAT 0 g

CHOLESTEROL 6 mg

SODIUM 140 mg

CARBOHYDRATE 80 g
DIETARY FIBER 6 g
SUGARS 45 g

PROTEIN 18 g

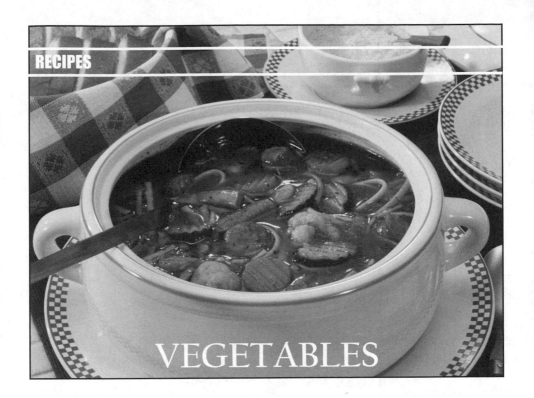

VEGETABLES

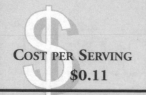

Cost per Serving
$0.11

CRUNCHY ORIENTAL COLESLAW

PREPARATION TIME
20 minutes

CHILLING TIME
1 hour

SERVINGS 16

SERVING SIZE
1/2 cup

EXCHANGES/ CHOICES
1 Vegetable
1 Fat

CALORIES 90
CALORIES FROM FAT 65

TOTAL FAT 7 g
SATURATED FAT 1 g
TRANS FAT 0 g

CHOLESTEROL 0 mg

SODIUM 190 mg

CARBOHYDRATE 6 g
DIETARY FIBER 1 g
SUGARS 2 g

PROTEIN 1 g

Try this coleslaw at your next picnic or potluck!

Dressing
1/3 cup canola oil
3 Tbsp white vinegar
2 tsp sugar
1/2 tsp salt
1/2 tsp ground black pepper
Seasoning packet from Oriental Ramen noodles

Salad
1 lb green cabbage, shredded
6 green onions, chopped
1 3-oz package Oriental Ramen noodles, crumbled
1/3 cup dry roasted sunflower seeds

1. In a small jar, combine dressing ingredients. Place lid tightly on jar and shake to combine. Dressing flavor is enhanced if made ahead and chilled in the refrigerator for about 1 hour before tossing with salad.

2. In a large bowl, combine salad ingredients. Toss dressing with salad and serve immediately to maintain crunchiness.

Marinated Confetti Vegetable Salad

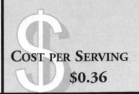

Cost per Serving
$0.36

The marinade lends a mild tanginess to this colorful and crunchy salad that incorporates tomatoes and cucumbers fresh from the garden.

Marinade
3 Tbsp white wine vinegar
1 1/2 tsp corn oil
1 tsp Dijon mustard
1 tsp (or 1 clove) minced garlic
1/4 tsp salt
1/8 tsp ground black pepper

Salad
1 15.25-oz can no salt added white corn, drained and rinsed
1 medium (approximately 5 oz) tomato, diced
1 medium (approximately 4 oz) cucumber, peeled and diced

1. Place marinade ingredients in a jar, cover tightly with lid, and shake to blend.

2. Combine corn, tomato, and cucumber in serving dish. Pour marinade over vegetables and toss to coat.

3. Cover and refrigerate for 1 hour to allow flavors to blend—stir twice while chilling.

Preparation Time
15 minutes

Chilling Time
1 hour

Servings 6

Serving Size
1/2 cup

Exchanges/Choices
2 Vegetable

Calories 55
Calories from Fat 20

Total Fat 2 g
Saturated Fat <1 g
Trans Fat 0 g

Cholesterol 0 mg

Sodium 125 mg

Carbohydrate 8 g
Dietary Fiber 2 g
Sugars 5 g

Protein 2 g

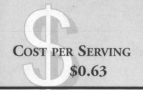

TOMATO SALAD SURPRISE

PREPARATION TIME
30 minutes

SERVINGS 10

SERVING SIZE
1/2 cup

EXCHANGES/CHOICES
1/2 Starch
1 Vegetable
1 Fat

CALORIES 105
CALORIES FROM FAT 30

TOTAL FAT 4 g
SATURATED FAT <1 g
TRANS FAT 0 g

CHOLESTEROL 0 mg

SODIUM 200 mg

CARBOHYDRATE 16 g
DIETARY FIBER 2 g
SUGARS 3 g

PROTEIN 3 g

The surprise ingredient in this salad is French bread cubes. Day-old French bread works best. If the bread is not very dry, bake it in the oven at 350ºF for 5 minutes before cubing.

5 large, juicy, cold, ripe tomatoes, peeled (approximately 2 1/2 lbs total)
2 Tbsp corn oil
1 Tbsp red wine vinegar
2 tsp (or 2 cloves) minced garlic
1/4 tsp salt
3 cups French bread cubes, crust removed
1 Tbsp chopped fresh parsley

1. Dice two tomatoes into bite-sized pieces and place in a serving dish. Put remaining three tomatoes in food processor and pulse until tomatoes are a coarse puree (you may also mash the tomatoes by hand).

2. Add puree, oil, vinegar, garlic, and salt to diced tomatoes; stir well. Toss bread cubes into tomato mixture, sprinkle with parsley, and serve immediately.

Feisty French Onion Soup

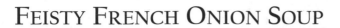

Cost per Serving
$0.62

This soup is just as flavorful reheated!

3 large onions (approximately 1 1/2 lbs total), thinly sliced
and separated into rings
5 1/2 cups (3 14.5-oz cans) 50% reduced-sodium beef
broth, fat removed
1 Tbsp Worcestershire sauce
1/4 tsp salt
1/8 tsp ground black pepper
6 1-inch slices French bread, lightly toasted
1/3 cup shredded part-skim mozzarella cheese

1. In a 4-or-5 quart saucepan, sauté onion in 1 cup beef
   broth over high heat until slightly tender (about 5
   minutes)—stir periodically.

2. Add remaining broth, Worcestershire sauce, salt, and
   pepper. Simmer covered over medium heat for 20
   minutes.

3. Place toasted bread on baking sheet and sprinkle with
   cheese. Broil 5 inches from heat source for 2 minutes
   or until cheese melts. Cut each piece of toast into 3
   strips.

4. Pour soup into 6 bowls and top each with 3 strips of
   cheese toast.

Preparation Time
10 minutes

Cooking Time
30 minutes

Servings 6

Serving Size
1 cup

Exchanges/Choices
1 Starch
2 Vegetable
1/2 Fat

Calories 460
Calories from Fat 20

Total Fat 2 g
Saturated Fat <1 g
Trans Fat 0 g

Cholesterol 5 mg

Sodium 745 mg

Carbohydrate 26 g
Dietary Fiber 2 g
Sugars 5 g

Protein 7 g

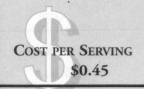

FAVORITE VEGETABLE SOUP

PREPARATION TIME
25 minutes

COOKING TIME
1 1/2 hours

SERVINGS 14

SERVING SIZE
1 cup

EXCHANGES/CHOICES
1 Starch
1 Vegetable

CALORIES 115
CALORIES FROM FAT 10

TOTAL FAT 1 g
SATURATED FAT <1 g
TRANS FAT 0 g

CHOLESTEROL 10 mg

SODIUM 130 mg

CARBOHYDRATE 20 g
DIETARY FIBER 4 g
SUGARS 6 g

PROTEIN 7 g

Vegetable soup is a great way to use leftover vegetables and even meat—replace each can of vegetable listed in the recipe with approximately 2 cups of that same vegetable from your leftovers. Also, you can replace ground chuck with 1/2 lb leftover shredded roast beef.

1/2 lb ground chuck
7 cups peeled, chopped fresh tomatoes or 2 28-oz cans
    no salt added diced tomatoes
4 cups water
1 14.5-oz can no salt added cut green beans, drained and
    rinsed
1 15-oz can no salt added peas, drained and rinsed
1 15.25-oz can no salt added corn, drained and rinsed
2 medium carrots (3 oz each), peeled and chopped
3 medium potatoes (5 oz each), peeled and diced
1 medium onion (5 oz), diced
1/4 cup dry rice
1/8 tsp ground black pepper
1/8 tsp red pepper flakes
1/2 tsp salt
1/2 tsp garlic powder

1. Place ground chuck in a 2-gallon stockpot and brown over medium heat. Remove meat and drain it well. Wipe drippings from pot.

2. Return meat to stockpot, then add tomatoes and water. Bring to a simmer and cook, covered, until tomatoes are soft and a juicy broth is created, about 20 minutes.

3. Add remaining ingredients, cover, and continue cooking 60 additional minutes to allow flavors to blend.

GARDEN VEGETABLE SCRAMBLE

COST PER SERVING
$0.46

This makes a colorful side dish—or a meatless meal when served with a slice of Gran's Country-Style Corn Bread, p. 80!

3 cups shredded green cabbage
2 medium (approximately 5 oz each) ears corn, cut from cob
2 medium (approximately 5 oz each) zucchini, chopped
1 large (approximately 8 oz) onion, chopped
3 medium fresh banana peppers (approximately 4 oz total), seeded and chopped
3 large tomatoes (approximately 1 1/2 lb total), peeled and chopped
1/8 cup water
1 1/2 Tbsp corn oil
1/8 tsp red pepper flakes
1/2 tsp salt
1/8 tsp ground black pepper

1. Combine all ingredients in a large pan. Simmer, uncovered, over medium heat for 25 minutes, stirring periodically.

PREPARATION TIME
30 minutes

COOKING TIME
25 minutes

SERVINGS 12

SERVING SIZE
1/2 cup

EXCHANGES/CHOICES
2 Vegetable

CALORIES 55
CALORIES FROM FAT 20

TOTAL FAT 2 g
SATURATED FAT <1 g
TRANS FAT 0 g

CHOLESTEROL 0 mg

SODIUM 110 mg

CARBOHYDRATE 10 g
DIETARY FIBER 2 g
SUGARS 4 g

PROTEIN 2 g

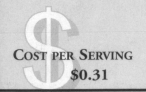

CAULIFLOWER SAUTÉ

PREPARATION TIME
10 minutes

COOKING TIME
15 minutes

SERVINGS 6

SERVING SIZE
1/2 cup

EXCHANGES/ CHOICES
1 Vegetable
1 Fat

CALORIES 55
CALORIES FROM FAT 40

TOTAL FAT 5 g
SATURATED FAT 1 g
TRANS FAT 0 g

CHOLESTEROL 0 mg

SODIUM 145 mg

CARBOHYDRATE 3 g
DIETARY FIBER 1 g
SUGARS 1 g

PROTEIN 1 g

Garlic's mellow taste is a remarkable complement to cauliflower in this recipe.

1 head (approximately 2 lb) cauliflower cut into
    bite-sized florets
2 Tbsp light margarine
1 1/2 tsp corn oil
1 tsp (or 1 clove) minced garlic
1/4 tsp salt
1/8 tsp ground black pepper
Paprika

1. Place cauliflower florets in a steamer basket above 2 inches boiling water. Cover and steam about 4 to 5 minutes or until cauliflower is crisp-tender when pierced with a fork. Remove from steam and keep warm.

2. Melt margarine in a large nonstick skillet. Add oil and garlic; sauté garlic over medium heat for 2 minutes.

3. Add steamed cauliflower and toss to coat. Continue sautéing for 5 additional minutes, stirring periodically.

4. Sprinkle with salt and pepper and toss. Place in serving dish and sprinkle with paprika.

GARLIC-PARMESAN MUSHROOMS

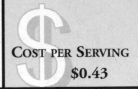

This easy appetizer is just bursting with flavor!

1 lb mushrooms, cleaned and stems removed
3 Tbsp light stick margarine, melted
1/4 tsp garlic salt
Cooking spray
1/8 cup grated Parmesan cheese
Paprika

1. Preheat broiler. Place cleaned mushrooms in a bowl. Combine margarine and garlic salt, then drizzle over mushrooms. Gently toss mushrooms to coat.

2. Spray a 9 × 13-inch baking sheet with sides (or a 9 × 13-inch pan) with cooking spray. Place mushrooms on baking sheet, stem-side up. Sprinkle with cheese, then lightly with paprika.

3. Broil 5 inches from heat source (crack oven door) for 5 minutes or until cheese is slightly melted. Serve immediately.

PREPARATION TIME
10 minutes

BROILING TIME
5 minutes

SERVINGS 8

SERVING SIZE
4 mushrooms

EXCHANGES/ CHOICES
1 Fat

CALORIES 50
CALORIES FROM FAT 35

TOTAL FAT 4 g
SATURATED FAT 1 g
TRANS FAT 0 g

CHOLESTEROL 1 mg

SODIUM 90 mg

CARBOHYDRATE 2 g
DIETARY FIBER 1 g
SUGARS 1 g

PROTEIN 2 g

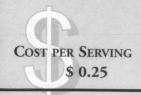

Cost per Serving
$ 0.25

Southern-Style Green Beans

Preparation Time
15 minutes

Cooking Time
1 hour, 40 minutes

Servings 6

Serving Size
1/2 cup

Exchanges/Choices
1 Vegetable
1/2 Fat

Calories 45
Calories from Fat 15

Total Fat 2 g
Saturated Fat <1 g
Trans Fat 0 g

Cholesterol 0 mg

Sodium 220 mg

Carbohydrate 7 g
Dietary Fiber 2 g
Sugars 2 g

Protein 1 g

Beef bouillon and onions lend southern flavor without the fat that traditional bacon or ham hocks add.

1 lb fresh green beans
2 1/2 cups water
2 tsp corn oil
2 cubes reduced-sodium beef bouillon
1/4 cup (approximately 2 1/2 oz) finely diced onion
1/8 tsp salt

1. Remove strings from green beans, then break beans into bite-sized pieces. Wash beans and place in 2-quart pan. Add water, oil, bouillon cubes, and onion. Bring to a simmer.

2. Cover and cook for 30 minutes or until beans are tender when pierced with a fork; stir periodically. Add salt, stir, and continue cooking an additional 60 minutes—most of the liquid should evaporate, and the beans should be very tender.

BROCCOLI ITALIANO

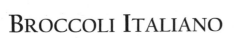

Italian dressing gives a nice zing to broccoli that's cooked just right—tender, but still a little crisp!

1 lb fresh (or thawed frozen) broccoli florets
1/4 cup fat-free Italian salad dressing

1. Place broccoli florets in steamer basket above 2 inches boiling water. Cover and steam 4 minutes or until broccoli is bright green and crisp-tender when pierced with a fork.
2. Remove from steam and place broccoli in serving dish. Drizzle with Italian dressing and toss to coat. Serve immediately.

PREPARATION TIME
5 minutes

COOKING TIME
4 minutes

SERVINGS 8

SERVING SIZE
1/2 cup

EXCHANGES/ CHOICES
1 Vegetable

CALORIES 20
CALORIES FROM FAT 0

TOTAL FAT 0 g
SATURATED FAT 0 g
TRANS FAT 0 g

CHOLESTEROL 0 mg

SODIUM 95 mg

CARBOHYDRATE 4 g
DIETARY FIBER 2 g
SUGARS 2 g

PROTEIN 2 g

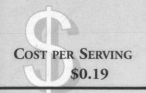

COST PER SERVING
$0.19

SQUASH MEDLEY

PREPARATION TIME
15 minutes

COOKING TIME
30 minutes

SERVINGS 14

SERVING SIZE
1/2 cup

EXCHANGES/CHOICES
1 Vegetable

CALORIES 25
CALORIES FROM FAT 15

TOTAL FAT 2 g
SATURATED FAT <1 g
TRANS FAT <1 g

CHOLESTEROL 0 mg

SODIUM 60 mg

CARBOHYDRATE 3 g
DIETARY FIBER 1 g
SUGARS 2 g

PROTEIN 1 g

Fresh squash should be heavy and firm, with a thin skin that can be punctured easily. If only hard-skinned squash is available, it should be peeled and seeded before cooking.

3 medium (approximately 1 lb) yellow summer squash, sliced 1/4 inch thick
3 medium (approximately 1 lb) zucchini squash, sliced 1/4 inch thick
1 medium (approximately 5 oz) onion, sliced 1/.8 inch thick and separated into rings
6 cups water (just enough to cover squash)
2 Tbsp light margarine
1/4 tsp salt
1/8 tsp ground black pepper
1/8 tsp garlic powder

1. Combine all ingredients in a 4-quart saucepan.

2. Cook uncovered over medium-high heat for 30 minutes or until vegetables are tender—if desired, may continue cooking to allow extra liquid to evaporate.

TASTY COOKED GREENS

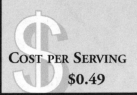

COST PER SERVING
$0.49

Use mustard, turnip, kale, or collard greens in this recipe.

2 lb fresh, tender greens
2 tsp corn oil
1/2 cup chopped onion
1 1/4 cups water
1 cube reduced-sodium chicken bouillon
1/4 tsp salt
1 tsp sugar
Dash Tabasco sauce

1. Remove stems and any yellowed leaves from greens, then rinse greens well and drain.

2. Heat oil in a large pot over medium heat. Add onion and sauté until onion is tender.

3. Add greens, water, and bouillon to the pot. Cover and bring to a boil. Reduce heat to low and simmer for 30 minutes or until greens are tender, stirring occasionally.

4. Add salt, sugar, and Tabasco sauce. Toss well and simmer an additional 5 minutes. May be served with cider vinegar to bring out the best in the greens.

PREPARATION TIME
20 minutes

COOKING TIME
45 minutes

SERVINGS 12

SERVING SIZE
1/2 cup

EXCHANGES/CHOICES
1 Vegetable

CALORIES 30
CALORIES FROM FAT 10

TOTAL FAT 1 g
SATURATED FAT <1 g
TRANS FAT 0 g

CHOLESTEROL 0 mg

SODIUM 100 mg

CARBOHYDRATE 5 g
DIETARY FIBER 2 g
SUGARS 1 g

PROTEIN 1 g

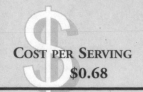

Cost per Serving
$0.68

Okra Jumble

Preparation Time
25 minutes

Cooking Time
35 minutes

Servings 10

Serving Size
1/2 cup

Exchanges/Choices
1/2 Starch
2 Vegetable

Calories 90
Calories from Fat 20

Total Fat 2 g
Saturated Fat <1 g
Trans Fat <1 g

Cholesterol 0 mg

Sodium 150 mg

Carbohydrate 16 g
Dietary Fiber 3 g
Sugars 5 g

Protein 3 g

Green, white, red, and yellow—okra, onion, tomatoes, and corn lend a jumble of colors and flavors to this simple dish!

2 Tbsp light tub margarine
1 cup chopped onion
3 cups sliced tender okra (approximately 1 1/2 lbs)
4 cups peeled, tomatoes (approximately 1 1/4 lbs)
    or 2 14.5-oz cans no salt added diced tomatoes
2 cups fresh corn (approximately 4 medium ears)
1/2 tsp salt
1/8 tsp ground black pepper
Dash Tabasco sauce

1. Melt margarine in a large pan, add onion, and cook over medium heat until onion is tender, about 5 minutes.

2. Add okra and cook 5 more minutes, stirring periodically.

3. Mix in tomatoes, corn, salt, pepper, and Tabasco. Cover and simmer over low heat for 25 minutes or until corn and okra are tender; stir occasionally.

LAYERED FIESTA SALAD

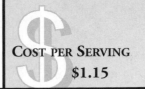
Homemade salsa adds a fresh touch to crunchy layers of Mexican flavor. Make the salsa first and let it chill while assembling the rest of the salad.

Salsa Dressing
1 10-oz can diced tomatoes with green chili peppers, drained
1 fresh jalapeno pepper (approximately 1 oz), seeded and cut into chunks (more or less to taste)
1 small (approximately 3 oz) onion, cut into chunks
1/2 of a 4.5-oz can chopped green chili peppers, drained
1/3 cup loosely packed fresh cilantro leaves, chopped
1 tsp (or 1 clove) minced garlic
Juice of 1/2 small lime

Salad
6 cups shredded lettuce
1/2 cup diced onion
1 11-oz can no salt added whole kernel corn, drained
1 medium (approximately 5 oz) green pepper, chopped
2 medium (approximately 5 oz each) tomatoes, diced
1/2 cup (approximately 2 oz) shredded cheddar cheese
1/2 cup crushed baked corn chips

1. In a food processor, combine diced tomatoes with green chili peppers, jalapeno, and onion. Process until desired texture. Transfer to a bowl and stir in green chili peppers, cilantro, garlic, and lime juice. Refrigerate 1 hour to allow flavors to blend.

2. Line a serving platter with shredded lettuce. Layer onion, corn, green pepper, and tomatoes. Drizzle salsa over salad and top with cheese and corn chips.

PREPARATION TIME
25 minutes

CHILLING TIME
1 hour

SERVINGS 6

SERVING SIZE
1 cup

EXCHANGES/CHOICES
1/2 Starch
2 Vegetable
1 Fat

CALORIES 129
CALORIES FROM FAT 36

TOTAL FAT 4 g
SATURATED FAT 2 g
TRANS FAT 0 g

CHOLESTEROL 10 mg

SODIUM 269 mg

CARBOHYDRATE 19 g
DIETARY FIBER 4 g
SUGARS 8 g

PROTEIN 6 g

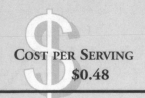

COST PER SERVING
$0.48

GREEN BEAN STIR-FRY

PREPARATION TIME
10 minutes

COOKING TIME
4 minutes

SERVINGS 6

SERVING SIZE
1/2 cup

EXCHANGES/CHOICES
1 Vegetable
1 Fat

CALORIES 80
CALORIES FROM FAT 49

TOTAL FAT 5 g
SATURATED FAT <1 g
TRANS FAT 0 g

CHOLESTEROL 0 mg

SODIUM 2 mg

CARBOHYDRATE 7 g
DIETARY FIBER 3 g
SUGARS 2 g

PROTEIN 3 g

Quick and crunchy!

1 lb fresh string beans, ends removed
1 Tbsp canola oil
1 tsp tomato-basil-garlic seasoning
1 medium (approximately 5 oz) tomato, diced
1/4 cup finely chopped green onions
1/4 cup sliced almonds

1. Bring a large pot of water to a boil.

2. Add green beans, return to a boil, and cook 1 minute. The beans will still be crisp. Drain, but don't rinse.

3. In a large skillet or wok, add oil. Heat until very hot (the skillet is ready when a drop of water sizzles in the oil). Add beans and cook 1 minute, turning often with a spatula. Sprinkle in seasoning, tomato, green onion, and almonds. Turn beans and nuts often to coat with oil and spices.

4. Cook about 2 minutes more or until beans and nuts are slightly browned.

Delicious Dill-Walnut Carrots

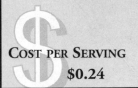
Cost per Serving
$0.24

A simple and tasty twist on cooked carrots.

3 cups grated carrots (approximately 14 oz)
1 Tbsp light margarine
1/8 tsp salt
1/2 tsp dill weed
2 Tbsp toasted chopped walnuts

1. Fill a saucepan with 1 inch of water, add carrots, and bring to a boil over high heat. Cover and cook 5–7 minutes, or until crisp-tender when pierced with a fork. Drain well.

2. Add margarine and sprinkle with salt and dill, then toss to coat.

3. Top with walnuts.

Preparation Time
10 minutes

Cooking Time
10–12 minutes

Servings 5

Serving Size
1/2 cup

Exchanges/Choices
1 Vegetable
1/2 Fat

Calories 59
Calories from Fat 29

Total Fat 3 g
Saturated Fat <1 g
Trans Fat 0 g

Cholesterol 0 mg

Sodium 128 mg

Carbohydrate 7 g
Dietary Fiber 2 g
Sugars 3 g

Protein 1 g

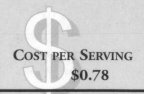

Cost per Serving
$0.78

Italian Stuffed Zucchini

Preparation Time
40 minutes

Cooking Time
40–45 minutes

Standing Time
1 hour

Servings 10

Serving Size
1/2 zucchini

Exchanges/Choices
2 Vegetable
1/2 Starch
1/2 Fat

Calories 109
Calories from Fat 37

Total Fat 4 g
Saturated Fat 1 g
Trans Fat 0 g

Cholesterol 4 mg

Sodium 144 mg

Carbohydrate 15 g
Dietary Fiber 3 g
Sugars 5 g

Protein 5 g

Double the salsa and enjoy it with baked tortilla chips.

Salsa
2 large tomatoes (1 lb total), seeded and chopped
3 Tbsp chopped fresh basil
1 Tbsp chopped fresh parsley
1 tsp grated lemon zest
1 clove minced garlic
Salt and pepper to taste
1 tsp olive oil

Zucchini
5 medium zucchini (approximately 1 1/2 lb total)
1 tsp olive oil
Cooking spray
2 Tbsp chopped fresh basil
3 Tbsp chopped fresh parsley
1 clove minced garlic
1 1/2 cups soft bread crumbs, lightly toasted (3 slices
   bread)
Salt and pepper to taste
1/4 cup shredded Parmesan cheese
1/2 cup fat-free 50% reduced-sodium chicken broth

1. Place all salsa ingredients in a bowl and stir to mix
   well. Let stand at room temperature 1 hour to allow
   flavors to blend. Preheat oven to 350°F.

2. Cut the stem ends off of zucchini and slice a thin
   layer off the tops lengthwise. If necessary, trim the
   bottoms so that the zucchini stand level; reserve
   trimmings.

3. Scoop out the zucchini flesh using a spoon or melon
   scoop, leaving 1/4-inch-thick shells. Coarsely chop the
   reserved trimmings and flesh.

4. Place zucchini shells in a large pan and fill with water to cover zucchini. Cover and bring to a boil; cook shells for 2 minutes.

5. Drain, rinse in cold water, then turn shells upside down to drain on paper towels.

6. Heat oil in a nonstick skillet coated with cooking spray over medium heat. Saute chopped zucchini for 5 minutes, or until tender. Stir in basil, parsley, and garlic and cook for 1 additional minute.

7. Transfer to a medium bowl and stir in bread crumbs and salt and pepper to taste.

8. Pack mixture into shells and place in a 9 x 13-inch baking dish. Pour chicken broth over stuffed zucchini. Cover and bake for 25–30 minutes, or until tender when pierced with a fork. Drain off remaining chicken broth and discard.

9. Sprinkle tops of stuffed zucchini with Parmesan cheese and spoon salsa over.

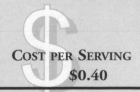

COST PER SERVING
$0.40

COTTAGE CHEESE AND GARDEN VEGGIE SALAD

PREPARATION TIME
15 minutes

SERVINGS 7

SERVING SIZE
1/2 cup

EXCHANGES/CHOICES
1 Vegetable
1 Very Lean Meat

CALORIES 44
CALORIES FROM FAT 1

TOTAL FAT 0 g
SATURATED FAT 0 g
TRANS FAT 0 g

CHOLESTEROL 3 mg

SODIUM 180 mg

CARBOHYDRATE 4 g
DIETARY FIBER 1 g
SUGARS 2 g

PROTEIN 7 g

Chopped cherry or grape tomatoes in place of a medium tomato work equally well in this salad.

12 oz fat-free cottage cheese
1 medium tomato (approximately 6 oz), seeded and chopped
1 medium cucumber (approximately 8 oz), peeled and diced
3 green onions, chopped
1/2 tsp dill weed
1/8 tsp black pepper

1. Combine all ingredients in a medium bowl and stir gently to mix. Allow flavors to blend by chilling 30 minutes before serving.

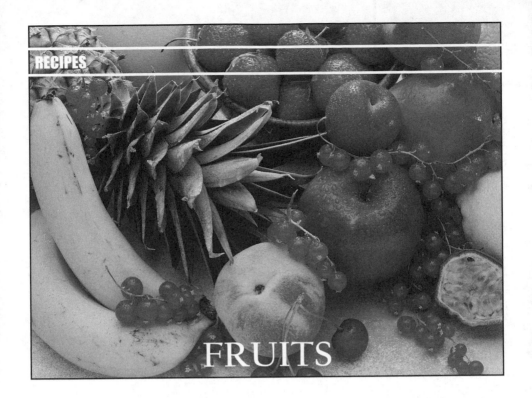

FRUITS

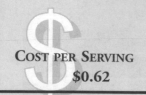

STRAWBERRY RIBBON SUPREME

PREPARATION TIME
25 minutes

CHILLING TIME
30 minutes

SERVINGS 9

SERVING SIZE
1 square

EXCHANGES/CHOICES
1 Fruit
1/2 Milk
1/2 Fat

CALORIES 135
CALORIES FROM FAT 25

TOTAL FAT 3 g
SATURATED FAT 2 g
TRANS FAT 0 g

CHOLESTEROL 15 mg

SODIUM 135 mg

CARBOHYDRATE 17 g
DIETARY FIBER 2 g
SUGARS 12 g

PROTEIN 7 g

This colorful creation is delicious served as a salad or a dessert.

2 0.3-oz packages sugar-free strawberry gelatin
1 2/3 cups boiling water
1 10-oz package unsweetened frozen strawberries, sliced
2 medium (approximately 6 oz each) bananas, peeled and sliced
1 15.25-oz can crushed pineapple in juice, drained well
4 oz reduced-fat cream cheese, softened
3 packets Aspartame artificial sweetener
2 cups fat-free sour cream

1. In a large bowl, dissolve gelatin in boiling water. Add frozen strawberries and stir until berries are thawed. Add bananas; then place gelatin in refrigerator for 5 minutes or until gelatin is slightly thickened. Remove from refrigerator and stir in drained pineapple.

2. Spoon half of gelatin mixture into a 9 × 9-inch pan and refrigerate 10 minutes. Leave remaining gelatin out of refrigerator.

3. Meanwhile, place cream cheese and Aspartame in a mixing bowl, and beat with an electric mixer until light and fluffy. Add sour cream and beat until mixture is smooth.

4. Remove gelatin from refrigerator and cover with cream cheese/sour cream mixture. Spoon remaining gelatin over and return to refrigerator. Chill until firm (about 30 minutes), then slice into 9 servings.

Fruit Fantasia

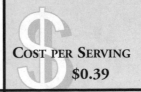

Cost per Serving
$0.39

Delight friends and family with this colorful salad or dessert! If chilling for more than 30 minutes, leave out the bananas, then toss them in just before serving.

2 medium (approximately 6 oz each) bananas, peeled and sliced
2 1/4 cups sliced fresh strawberries
1 20-oz can pineapple tidbits in juice, drained and with juice reserved
1 15-oz can sliced peaches in juice, drained and with juice reserve
1 tsp sugar-free Tang drink mix
1 0.9-oz package sugar-free vanilla instant pudding mix

1. In a large serving dish, combine bananas, strawberries, pineapple, and peaches; set aside.

2. In a separate bowl, combine reserved pineapple juice, Tang mix, and pudding mix. Mix well using a wire whisk—it will be thick.

3. Spoon pudding mixture over fruit and toss gently to coat. May thin with reserved peach juice as desired. Chill 30 minutes before serving.

Preparation Time
15 minutes

Chilling Time
30 minutes

Servings 12

Serving Size
1/2 cup

Exchanges/Choices
1 Fruit

Calories 75
Calories from Fat 0

Total Fat 0 g
Saturated Fat 0 g
Trans Fat 0 g

Cholesterol 0 mg

Sodium 105 mg

Carbohydrate 19 g
Dietary Fiber 2 g
Sugars 13 g

Protein 1 g

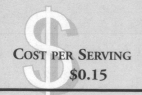

CINNAMON-GLAZED BANANAS

PREPARATION TIME
15 minutes

SERVINGS 6

SERVING SIZE
1/2 banana

EXCHANGES/CHOICES
1 Fruit
1/2 Carbohydrate
1/2 Fat

CALORIES 125
CALORIES FROM FAT 30

TOTAL FAT 4 g
SATURATED FAT 1 g
TRANS FAT 0 g

CHOLESTEROL 0 mg

SODIUM 35 mg

CARBOHYDRATE 24 g
DIETARY FIBER 2 g
SUGARS 16 g

PROTEIN 1 g

Cinnamon and orange juice complement the natural sweetness of bananas in this simple dessert.

3 medium (approximately 6 oz each) bananas
2 Tbsp light tub margarine
2 Tbsp packed light brown sugar
3 Tbsp thawed unsweetened orange juice concentrate
1 tsp vanilla extract
1/4 tsp ground cinnamon
6 Tbsp frozen fat-free whipped topping

1. Peel bananas and cut in half lengthwise, then cut in half crosswise.

2. Melt margarine in a large nonstick skillet over medium heat. Add brown sugar, orange juice concentrate, vanilla extract, and cinnamon. Heat for 30 seconds while stirring constantly.

3. Add banana quarters and cook for 1 minute. Gently turn banana quarters and cook 1 more minute.

4. Remove bananas to individual serving dishes, spoon sauce over, and top each serving with 1 Tbsp frozen whipped topping.

Fresh Pears
with Berries and "Cream"

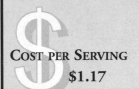

Cost per Serving
$1.17

Enjoy fresh, juicy pears nestled in a rich tasting "cream" created by combining vanilla yogurt, orange juice, and honey.

1 6-oz container sugar-free, fat-free vanilla yogurt
1 Tbsp unsweetened orange juice
1/4 cup honey
6 pears (approximately 2 lb total)
1/2 cup fresh blueberries
1/2 cup fresh raspberries
Ground cinnamon

1. In a medium bowl, whisk together yogurt, orange juice, and honey; set aside.

2. Peel, core, and thinly slice each pear lengthwise. Arrange pear slices on six plates.

3. Spoon yogurt mixture over each pear, and sprinkle with both blueberries and raspberries. Sprinkle lightly with cinnamon and serve immediately.

Preparation Time
15 minutes

Servings 6

Serving Size
1 pear

Exchanges/Choices
2 1/2 Fruit

Calories 173
Calories from Fat 9

Total Fat 1 g
Saturated Fat <1 g
Trans Fat 0 g

Cholesterol 1 mg

Sodium 32 mg

Carbohydrate 39 g
Dietary Fiber 5 g
Sugars 19 g

Protein 2 g

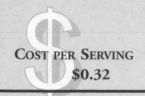

COST PER SERVING
$0.32

FROZEN HAWAIIAN FRUIT SALAD

PREPARATION TIME
20 minutes

FREEZING TIME
2 hours

STANDING TIME
20 minutes

SERVINGS 24

SERVING SIZE
1 baking cup

EXCHANGES/ CHOICES
1 Fruit

CALORIES 70
CALORIES FROM FAT 0

TOTAL FAT 0 g
SATURATED FAT 0 g
TRANS FAT 0 g

CHOLESTEROL 0 mg

SODIUM 0 mg

CARBOHYDRATE 17 g
DIETARY FIBER 1 g
SUGARS 14 g

PROTEIN 1 g

This can also be served as a light dessert.

1 20-oz can crushed pineapple in juice
Water
18 oz frozen unsweetened pineapple-orange-banana juice
    concentrate, thawed
2 medium (approximately 6 oz each) bananas, peeled,
    quartered lengthwise, and diced into bite-sized chunks
1 15-oz can mandarin oranges, drained and rinsed, each
    slice cut in half
24 paper baking cups
Lettuce leaves (optional)

1. Drain pineapple using a sieve, reserving juice in a 2-cup
   liquid measuring cup. Add water to reserved juice to
   make 1 1/2 cups liquid.

2. Pour liquid into a large mixing bowl. Add pineapple,
   thawed juice concentrate, bananas, and mandarin
   oranges; mix well.

3. Line muffin tins with paper baking cups. Spoon fruit
   mixture into paper baking cups (fill each 3/4 full).
   Cover tightly with plastic wrap, and freeze 2 hours or
   until firm.

4. Before serving, remove desired number of cups from
   freezer and let stand 20 minutes to soften slightly.
   Remove salad from cups and serve on a lettuce leaf if
   desired.

Apple-Prune Spread

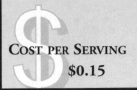
Cost per Serving
$0.15

This spread is delicious slathered on toast, waffles, or pancakes. Packaged in a pleasing container, this makes a nice gift.

4 large (approximately 8 oz each) Granny Smith apples, peeled, cored, and sliced
1 12-oz package pitted prunes
1 cup unsweetened apple juice
1 1/2 tsp cinnamon
1/2 tsp allspice
1/2 tsp lemon juice

1. Combine apples, prunes, apple juice, cinnamon, and allspice in a 2-quart saucepan. Bring to a boil over high heat. Reduce heat until fruit is at a simmer and cook for 10 minutes.

2. Uncover and continue cooking, stirring periodically, until fruits are cooked down and most of liquid is absorbed, about 15 minutes. Remove from heat and add lemon juice.

3. Beat with an electric mixer on high speed until smooth. May serve while warm or transfer to storage container, cover tightly, and store in refrigerator—will keep about three weeks.

Preparation Time
10 minutes

Cooking Time
30 minutes

Servings 32

Serving Size
2 Tbsp

Exchanges/ Choices
1 Fruit

Calories 44
Calories from Fat 0

Total Fat 0 g
Saturated Fat 0 g
Trans Fat 0 g

Cholesterol 0 mg

Sodium 4 mg

Carbohydrate 10 g
Dietary Fiber 1 g
Sugars 4 g

Protein 1 g

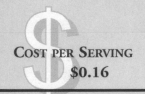

COST PER SERVING
$0.16

TROPICAL SLUSHY

PREPARATION TIME
5 minutes

SERVINGS 4

SERVING SIZE
1 cup

EXCHANGES/CHOICES
1 Fruit

CALORIES 75
CALORIES FROM FAT 0

TOTAL FAT 0 g
SATURATED FAT 0 g
TRANS FAT 0 g

CHOLESTEROL 0 mg

SODIUM 0 mg

CARBOHYDRATE 19 g
DIETARY FIBER 1 g
SUGARS 15 g

PROTEIN 1 g

Banana, pineapple juice, and orange juice contribute a tropical flavor to this icy drink.

1 medium (approximately 6 oz) ripe banana, peeled
1/2 cup unsweetened pineapple juice
1 cup unsweetened orange juice
1 tsp fresh-squeezed lemon juice
1/2 tsp vanilla extract
4 tsp Splenda granular
4 cups ice cubes

1. Combine all ingredients in a blender and blend on high until smooth and slushy. Serve immediately.

BERRY AND BANANA BLEND

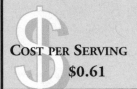
COST PER SERVING
$0.61

Use leftover blueberries from the Fresh Pears with Berries and "Cream," p. 127.

1/2 cup fat-free milk
4 ice cubes
1/2 cup fresh or unsweetened frozen blueberries, thawed
1 medium (approximately 6 oz) ripe banana, peeled
4 oz sugar-free, fat-free vanilla yogurt
1 tsp vanilla extract
1/8 tsp cinnamon

1. Combine milk and ice cubes in a blender, cover, and whip until icy smooth.

2. Add fruit and whip again.

3. Add yogurt, vanilla extract, and cinnamon, then blend until combined. Serve immediately.

PREPARATION TIME
10 minutes

SERVINGS 2

SERVING SIZE
1 cup

EXCHANGES/CHOICES
1 1/2 Fruit
1/2 Milk

CALORIES 125
CALORIES FROM FAT 0

TOTAL FAT 0 g
SATURATED FAT <1 g
TRANS FAT 0 g

CHOLESTEROL 0 mg

SODIUM 60 mg

CARBOHYDRATE 27 g
DIETARY FIBER 3 g
SUGARS 17 g

PROTEIN 5 g

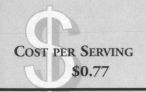

COST PER SERVING
$0.77

PERSONAL FRUIT PARFAIT

PREPARATION TIME
5–7 minutes

SERVINGS 1

SERVING SIZE
1 parfait

EXCHANGES/CHOICES
1 1/2 Fruit
1/2 Milk

CALORIES 119
CALORIES FROM FAT 46

TOTAL FAT 5 g
SATURATED FAT <1 g
TRANS FAT 0 g

CHOLESTEROL 1 mg

SODIUM 32 mg

CARBOHYDRATE 17 g
DIETARY FIBER 2 g
SUGARS 13 g

PROTEIN 3 g

If you wish to make this colorful parfait ahead, dip the apple slices in lemon juice before assembling the parfait to prevent browning.

1/3 medium (approximately 5 oz) apple, sliced
1/4 cup no sugar added, fat-free vanilla yogurt
1/8 cup green grapes
1/8 cup mandarin oranges canned in juice, drained
1 Tbsp toasted walnuts, crumbled

1. Layer the following in a clear 8- to 10-oz cup:
   Half of the apple slices
   1 Tbsp yogurt
   Grapes
   1 Tbsp yogurt
   Mandarin oranges
   1 Tbsp yogurt
   Remaining half of apple slices
   1 Tbsp yogurt

2. Sprinkle with toasted walnuts.

APPLE-RASPBERRY TEA SPARKLER

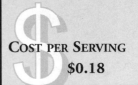
COST PER SERVING
$0.18

This sparkling tea with a light apple-raspberry flavor is sure to be a favorite at your next dinner party. Vary the flavor of juice used for an array of tea sparklers.

2 tea bags
1 1/2 cups boiling water
2 cups apple-raspberry 100% juice
Artificial sweetener to taste (optional)
1 1/2 cups club soda
Fresh mint and fresh raspberries for garnish (optional)

1. Place 2 tea bags in 1 1/2 cups boiling water and set aside to steep for 15 minutes.

2. Remove tea bags and pour tea concentrate into a pitcher. Add juice and artificial sweetener to taste. Stir to mix. May chill at this point if desired.

3. Stir in club soda right before serving.

4. Pour over ice and garnish with fresh mint and raspberries.

PREPARATION TIME
5 minutes

STANDING TIME
15 minutes

SERVINGS 5

SERVING SIZE
1 cup

EXCHANGES/ CHOICES
1 Fruit

CALORIES 44
CALORIES FROM FAT 2

TOTAL FAT 0 g
SATURATED FAT 0 g
TRANS FAT 0 g

CHOLESTEROL 0 mg

SODIUM 20 mg

CARBOHYDRATE 11 g
DIETARY FIBER 0 g
SUGARS 10 g

PROTEIN 0 g

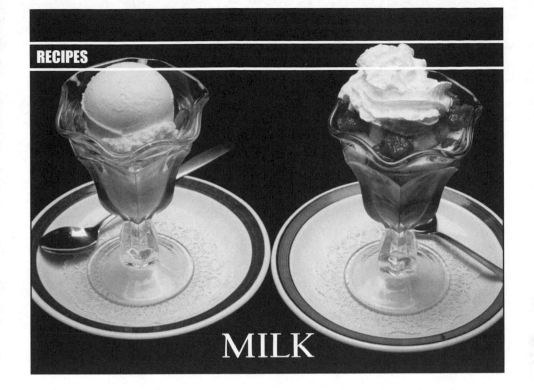

MILK

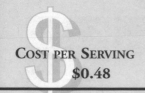

DO-IT-YOURSELF DRINKABLE YOGURT

PREPARATION TIME
5 minutes

SERVINGS 2 1/2

SERVING SIZE
1 cup

EXCHANGES/CHOICES
1 Fruit
1/2 Milk

CALORIES 95
CALORIES FROM FAT 1

TOTAL FAT 0 g
SATURATED FAT 0 g
TRANS FAT 0 g

CHOLESTEROL 3 mg

SODIUM 74 mg

CARBOHYDRATE 20 g
DIETARY FIBER 0 g
SUGARS 16 g

PROTEIN 4 g

An inexpensive alternative (for kids of all ages) to pricey bottles of drinkable yogurt. Use different fruit juices to vary the flavor of the yogurt.

2 6-oz containers no sugar added, fat-free vanilla yogurt
1 cup 100% cherry fruit juice (such as Juicy Juice)
1/2 cup cold water
2–4 drops red food coloring (optional)

1. Combine all ingredients in a large bowl and whisk to mix well. Transfer to a pitcher with a lid, cover, and refrigerate.

2. Shake well before serving.

Purple Cow Pops

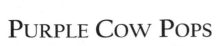

Cost per Serving
$0.32

Creamy grape pops—it can't get any easier than two ingredients!

3 6-oz containers no sugar added, fat-free vanilla yogurt
1/4 cup + 2 Tbsp unsweetened frozen grape juice
  concentrate, thawed

1. In a mixing bowl, combine yogurt and grape juice concentrate; stir well.

2. Pour into small frozen-pop molds or 5-oz wax-coated paper cups, filling 3/4 full, and freeze solid (about 2 hours). If using paper cups, partially freeze (about 1 hour), then insert wooden craft sticks. Tear off cups when frozen solid.

PREPARATION TIME
10 minutes

FREEZING TIME
2 hours

SERVINGS 5

SERVING SIZE
1 pop

EXCHANGES/ CHOICES
1/2 Fruit
1/2 Milk

CALORIES 75
CALORIES FROM FAT 0

TOTAL FAT 0 g
SATURATED FAT 0 g
TRANS FAT 0 g

CHOLESTEROL 0 mg

SODIUM 55 mg

CARBOHYDRATE 16 g
DIETARY FIBER 0 g
SUGARS 14 g

PROTEIN 3 g

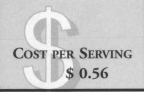

STRAWBERRY WHIP

PREPARATION TIME
10 minutes

SERVINGS 6

SERVING SIZE
1 cup

EXCHANGES/CHOICES
1/2 Milk
1 Carbohydrate

CALORIES 105
CALORIES FROM FAT 0

TOTAL FAT 0 g
SATURATED FAT 0 g
TRANS FAT 0 g

CHOLESTEROL 0 mg

SODIUM 60 mg

CARBOHYDRATE 20 g
DIETARY FIBER 1 g
SUGARS 9 g

PROTEIN 3 g

Use as a creamy, light dessert or as a dip for fresh fruit.

3 6-oz containers no sugar added, fat-free strawberry
    yogurt
1 8-oz container frozen fat-free whipped topping, thawed
1/2 cup crushed fresh or unsweetened thawed frozen
    strawberries
6 fresh strawberries for garnish

1. Place all ingredients in a large mixing bowl and whisk
   together. Cover and chill if not serving immediately.

2. Serve in individual glass dishes garnished with a
   fresh strawberry.

3. For a frosty dessert, pour into an 8 × 8-inch pan,
   freeze for 2 1/2 hours, thaw slightly, cut into 6 squares,
   and garnish each square with a fresh strawberry.

CARIBBEAN SUNRISE SMOOTHIE

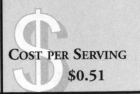
COST PER SERVING
$0.51

Put fruit in the freezer the night before so that you can whip this breakfast drink together quickly. Transfer pineapple to a covered plastic container before freezing. If the pineapple is frozen solid by morning, thaw slightly for a few seconds in the microwave.

1 small (approximately 5 oz) peeled, ripe banana, frozen
1 8-oz can crushed pineapple in juice, frozen until slushy
3 6-oz containers no sugar added, fat-free coconut cream pie yogurt
1/2 cup unsweetened orange juice

1. Place all ingredients in a blender and whip until smooth.

PREPARATION TIME
5 minutes

FREEZING TIME
6 hours

SERVINGS 4

SERVING SIZE
1 cup

EXCHANGES/CHOICES
1 Fruit
1/2 Milk

CALORIES 105
CALORIES FROM FAT 0

TOTAL FAT 0 g
SATURATED FAT 0 g
TRANS FAT 0 g

CHOLESTEROL 5 mg

SODIUM 60 mg

CARBOHYDRATE 23 g
DIETARY FIBER 1 g
SUGARS 18 g

PROTEIN 4 g

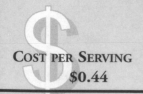

HOT CHOCOLATE WITH WHIPPED TOPPING AND PEPPERMINT

PREPARATION TIME
5–7 minutes

SERVINGS 1

SERVING SIZE
1 cup

EXCHANGES/CHOICES
1 Milk
1 Carbohydrate

CALORIES 150
CALORIES FROM FAT 15

TOTAL FAT 2 g
SATURATED FAT 1 g

TRANS FAT 0 g

CHOLESTEROL 5 mg

SODIUM 175 mg

CARBOHYDRATE 24 g
DIETARY FIBER 0 g
SUGARS 18 g

PROTEIN 9 g

The hint of peppermint pleasantly complements this steaming chocolate beverage.

1 Tbsp instant sugar-free chocolate milk mix
1 cup fat-free milk
2 Tbsp frozen "lite" whipped topping, thawed
1 red and white peppermint candy, crushed

1. Combine chocolate milk mix and milk in a small saucepan; whisk until mix is dissolved. Heat uncovered over medium heat until milk is hot; stir frequently to prevent scorching—do not boil.

2. Pour into a mug and top with whipped topping, then crushed peppermint.

Cinnamon-Honey Eggnog

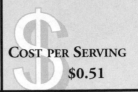

Cost per Serving
$0.51

Try garnishing each mug with a twist of orange peel and a sprinkle of cinnamon. Before measuring the honey for this recipe, try coating the measuring spoon with cooking spray to prevent the honey from sticking to it.

6 cups fat-free milk
1 cup liquid egg substitute
5 Tbsp honey
1 1/2 tsp vanilla extract
1/4 tsp ground cinnamon

1. Combine milk, egg substitute, and honey in a large pan, whisking well. Place over medium heat and cook for 15 minutes or until eggnog becomes frothy on top and bubbles gently. When eggnog becomes warm, whisk frequently to prevent scorching. Remove pan from heat.

2. Stir in vanilla extract and cinnamon. Chill eggnog at least 3 hours before serving—will thicken slightly upon chilling.

Preparation Time
5 minutes

Cooking Time
15 minutes

Chilling Time
3 hours

Servings 7

Serving Size
1 cup

Exchanges/Choices
1 Carbohydrate
1 Milk

Calories 145
Calories from Fat 0

Total Fat 0 g
Saturated Fat <1 g
Trans Fat 0 g

Cholesterol 5 mg

Sodium 180 mg

Carbohydrate 24 g
Dietary Fiber 0 g
Sugars 23 g

Protein 11 g

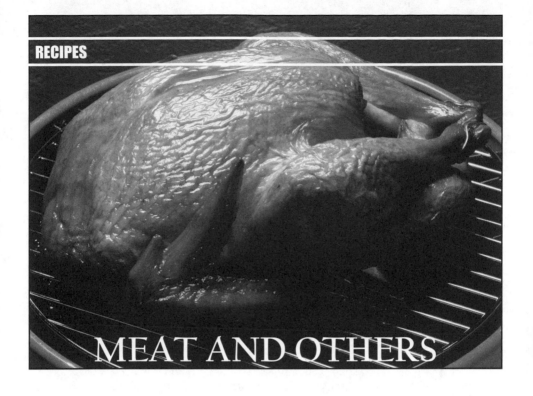

RECIPES

MEAT AND OTHERS

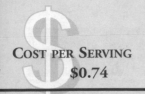

ITALIAN CHICKEN SKILLET

PREPARATION TIME
10 minutes

COOKING TIME
20 minutes

SERVINGS 4

SERVING SIZE
2/3 cup pasta
1 cup sauce

EXCHANGES/CHOICES
2 1/2 Starch
2 Lean Meat

CALORIES 260
CALORIES FROM FAT 30

TOTAL FAT 4 g
SATURATED FAT <1 g
TRANS FAT 0 g

CHOLESTEROL 35 mg

SODIUM 140 mg

CARBOHYDRATE 38 g
DIETARY FIBER 3 g
SUGARS 8 g

PROTEIN 20 g

Cutting up a whole chicken can be a challenge. You'll need a strong sturdy knife, a large cutting board, and kitchen or poultry shears. The chicken should yield eight pieces: 2 drumsticks, 2 thighs, 2 wings, and 2 breast halves.

Cooking spray
1 tsp corn oil
1 tsp (or 1 clove) minced garlic
1/4 cup diced onion
1 8-oz boneless, skinless chicken breast, diced into bite-sized pieces
1 7-oz can mushroom stems and pieces, drained and rinsed
1 small zucchini squash (approximately 3 oz), quartered lengthwise and diced into bite-sized pieces
1 14-oz jar reduced-sodium spaghetti sauce
1/2 cup water
1/8 tsp red pepper flakes
2 2/3 cups cooked pasta, cooked without added salt or oil

1. Coat a large nonstick skillet with cooking spray. Add oil and warm over medium heat. Add garlic and onion. Cook until onion turns clear (about 3 minutes), stirring frequently.

2. Add chicken and cook until no longer pink (about 7 minutes). Stir in mushrooms, zucchini, spaghetti sauce, water, and red pepper flakes.

3. Reduce heat to low, cover, and cook for 10 minutes, stirring periodically. Serve over hot pasta.

Marilyn's Spicy "Fried" Chicken

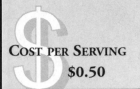
Cost per Serving
$0.50

This is a great recipe to use for planned-overs. Double the recipe and dice the extra cooked chicken, then toss with fresh lettuce, tomato, cucumber, mushrooms, onion, and low-fat dressing for a refreshing salad, or stuff it in a pita pocket for a sandwich with a twist.

3 egg whites
1 1-oz packet ranch-style salad dressing mix
1/2 tsp ground black pepper
3/4 cup dry unseasoned bread crumbs
5 6-oz boneless, skinless chicken breasts
Cooking spray
1 Tbsp corn oil

1. Preheat oven to 375°F.

2. Place egg whites in a large bowl and mix well with wire whisk. In a large zip-top plastic bag, combine salad dressing mix, pepper, and bread crumbs.

3. Dip each piece of chicken in egg whites to coat, then place in bag of seasonings and shake until well coated.

4. Lay chicken on baking sheet coated with cooking spray, and sprinkle with remaining seasoned crumbs.

5. Spray chicken with cooking spray, and bake for 20–25 minutes. Brush with corn oil, and bake 10 minutes longer or until chicken is tender and no longer pink.*

Before serving, reserve one breast if you want to prepare Southwestern Chicken Wrap-Ups this week.

Preparation Time
15 minutes

Baking Time
30–35 minutes

Servings 10

Serving Size
3 oz

Exchanges/Choices
1/2 Starch
3 Lean Meat

Calories 187
Calories from Fat 63

Total Fat 7 g
Saturated Fat 2 g
Trans Fat 0 g

Cholesterol 69 mg

Sodium 221 mg

Carbohydrate 7 g
Dietary Fiber <1 g
Sugars <1 g

Protein 24 g

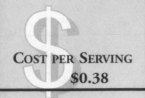

SOUTHWESTERN CHICKEN WRAP-UPS

PREPARATION TIME
20 minutes

SERVINGS 10

SERVING SIZE
1 wrap-up

EXCHANGES/CHOICES
2 Starch
1 Lean Meat

CALORIES 210
CALORIES FROM FAT 30

TOTAL FAT 4 g
SATURATED FAT <1 g
TRANS FAT 0 g

CHOLESTEROL 15 mg

SODIUM 420 mg

CARBOHYDRATE 33 g
DIETARY FIBER 5 g
SUGARS 3 g

PROTEIN 11 g

Combine small leftover amounts of rice, corn, black beans, and chicken for a delicious meal! Salsa and fat-free sour cream make tasty toppers for these wrap-ups.

Cooking spray
1/4 cup finely diced green pepper
1/4 cup finely diced onion
1 cup cooked white rice
1 cup corn or 1 8.75-oz can no salt added corn, drained
1/2 15-oz can black beans, drained and rinsed, or 1 cup
 cooked dried black beans
1 Tbsp Red Hot Sauce
1 breast from Marilyn's Spicy "Fried" Chicken
 or substitute 1 6-oz boneless, skinless grilled chicken
 breast, thinly sliced and warmed
10 7-inch whole-wheat flour tortillas, warmed
1/2 cup + 2 Tbsp salsa
Fat-free sour cream (optional)

1. In a small nonstick skillet coated with cooking spray, sauté green pepper and onion over medium heat until onion turns clear (about 3 minutes).

2. Add rice, corn, beans, and Red Hot Sauce to pepper and onion—toss to combine. Warm over medium-low heat for 5 minutes.

3. Divide rice mixture and chicken evenly among the 10 tortillas (approximately 1/3 cup filling per tortilla), spreading down the center. Roll up each tortilla, placing seam-side down on plate, and drizzle with 1 Tbsp salsa.

Oven-Barbecued Chicken

Cost per Serving $0.50

"Poultry is for the cook what canvas is for the painter." —Brillat-Savarin

1/4 cup white vinegar
1/4 cup water
1 Tbsp corn oil
1/2 cup ketchup
3 Tbsp Worcestershire sauce
2 Tbsp finely diced onion
2 Tbsp brown sugar (light or dark)
1/8 tsp garlic powder
2 tsp dry mustard
1/4 tsp salt
1/8 tsp coarse ground black pepper
4 6-oz boneless, skinless chicken breasts
Cooking spray

1. Preheat oven to 350°F. Combine all sauce ingredients in a small saucepan and simmer for 15 minutes over medium-low heat, stirring occasionally.

2. Place chicken in a 9 × 13-inch baking dish coated with cooking spray. Cover chicken evenly with 1 cup barbecue sauce.

3. Bake for 20–25 minutes, baste with remaining sauce, and cook another 5–10 minutes (or until chicken is tender and no longer pink).

Preparation Time
20 minutes

Baking Time
30–35 minutes

Servings 8

Serving Size
3 oz

Exchanges/Choices
1/2 Carbohydrate
3 Lean Meat

Calories 150
Calories from Fat 35

Total Fat 4 g
Saturated Fat <1 g
Trans Fat 0 g

Cholesterol 50 mg

Sodium 370 mg

Carbohydrate 9 g
Dietary Fiber 0 g
Sugars 7 g

Protein 19 g

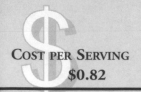

CLASSIC CHICKEN AND DUMPLINGS

PREPARATION TIME
25 minutes

COOKING TIME
1 hour

SERVINGS 8

SERVING SIZE
1 1/2 cups

EXCHANGES/CHOICES
2 1/2 Starch
2 Lean Meat

CALORIES 295
CALORIES FROM FAT 70

TOTAL FAT 8 g
SATURATED FAT 1 g
TRANS FAT 0 g

CHOLESTEROL 50 mg

SODIUM 705 mg

CARBOHYDRATE 36 g
DIETARY FIBER 1 g
SUGARS 5 g

PROTEIN 20 g

Cut up one whole chicken (about 4 lb)—you can use the breast to make Chinese Chicken Soup, p. 149.

1 cut-up chicken (about 4 lb)
3 quarts water
2 tsp sodium-free instant chicken bouillon granules
1 medium onion (approximately 5 oz), finely chopped
2 ribs celery, finely diced (1 cup diced)
1 carrot (approximately 3 oz), peeled and finely diced
1/4 tsp garlic powder
1/2 tsp salt
1/4 tsp ground black pepper
1 tsp dried parsley flakes
1/4 cup all-purpose flour
1 cup cold water
3 cups all-purpose reduced-fat baking mix
1 cup fat-free milk

1. Place chicken, 3 quarts water, bouillon, onion, celery, and carrot in a 2-gallon stockpot. Cover and bring to boil over high heat. Reduce heat to medium and cook for 30 minutes or until meat is tender and pulls away from the bone.

2. Remove chicken from broth. Skim fat from top of broth. Debone chicken. Discard skin and bones, shred meat, and return meat to broth.

3. Add garlic powder, salt, pepper, and parsley and return to boil over high heat.

4. In a liquid measuring cup, dissolve flour in 1 cup cold water, whisking well. Add to boiling liquid and stir until slightly thickened.

5. Place all-purpose baking mix and milk in a medium mixing bowl and stir to combine. Drop by tablespoons into boiling liquid. Reduce heat to medium, cover pot, and simmer for 20 minutes or until dumplings are fluffy; gently stir periodically.

CHINESE CHICKEN SOUP

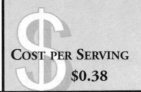

COST PER SERVING
$0.38

Cut up one whole chicken (about 4 lb)—use the breast in this soup and the remaining pieces to make Classic Chicken and Dumplings, p. 148.

1 whole chicken breast (approximately 12 oz total), skin removed
8 cups water
2 cubes reduced-sodium chicken bouillon
1/2 cup uncooked medium-grain rice
1 1/2 cups finely diced celery (3 ribs)
1 cup finely diced onion
1 7-oz can mushroom stems and pieces, drained
2 Tbsp reduced-sodium soy sauce
1/4 tsp garlic powder
1/8 tsp salt
1/8 tsp ground black pepper

1. In a 1-gallon stockpot, place chicken, water, and bouillon. Cover and bring to a boil over high heat. Simmer chicken about 20 minutes, or until no longer pink.

2. Remove chicken from liquid. Remove meat from the bone and shred it. Return shredded meat to liquid.

3. Add remaining ingredients and simmer uncovered over medium heat for 20 minutes or until rice is tender; stir periodically.

PREPARATION TIME
45 minutes

SERVINGS 9

SERVING SIZE
1 cup

EXCHANGES/CHOICES
1/2 Starch
1 Vegetable
1 Lean Meat

CALORIES 105
CALORIES FROM FAT 10

TOTAL FAT 1 g
SATURATED FAT <1 g
TRANS FAT 0 g

CHOLESTEROL 20 mg

SODIUM 345 mg

CARBOHYDRATE 14 g
DIETARY FIBER 1 g
SUGARS 2 g

PROTEIN 10 g

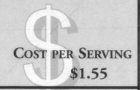

SESAME CHICKEN AND VEGETABLES

PREPARATION TIME
15 minutes

COOKING TIME
35–40 minutes

SERVINGS 6

SERVING SIZE
1 cup meat mixture
1/2 cup rice

EXCHANGES/CHOICES
2 Starch
2 Vegetable
1 Lean Meat

CALORIES 250
CALORIES FROM FAT 35

TOTAL FAT 4 g
SATURATED FAT <1 g

TRANS FAT 0 g

CHOLESTEROL 25 mg

SODIUM 560 mg

CARBOHYDRATE 37 g
DIETARY FIBER 4 g
SUGARS 4 g

This recipe incorporates canned chicken to simplify preparation and shorten cooking time.

1 cup uncooked medium-grain rice
1/2 head broccoli (approximately 8 oz)
1 Tbsp corn oil
2 carrots (approximately 3 oz each), peeled and cut into matchsticks
1 large onion (approximately 8 oz), coarsely chopped
1 7-oz can mushroom stems and pieces, drained
1 tsp (or 1 clove) minced garlic
1 10-oz can 96% fat-free chunk chicken in water, drained
1 cup fat-free 50% reduced-sodium chicken broth
2 Tbsp reduced-sodium soy sauce
1 tsp cornstarch
1/4 tsp ground ginger
1 tsp sesame seeds, lightly toasted

1. Cook rice according to package directions, omitting fat and salt.

2. Portion broccoli head into bite-sized florets. Peel broccoli stem and slice into bite-sized pieces.

3. In a large skillet, warm oil over high heat. Add broccoli, carrots, onion, mushrooms, and garlic. Cook, stirring frequently, for 3 minutes. Reduce heat to medium, add chicken, cover skillet, and cook until crisp-tender, about 4 minutes.

4. In a small bowl, combine broth, soy sauce, cornstarch, and ginger. Whisk until mixed. Pour into vegetable/chicken mixture and cook, stirring frequently, until sauce thickens slightly, about 1 minute. Cook an additional 2 minutes.

5. Spoon over cooked rice, sprinkle with toasted sesame seeds, and serve immediately.

Golden Roasted Turkey Breast

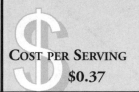
COST PER SERVING
$0.37

Turkey breast is excellent for a dinner party or a holiday meal. Leftovers make yummy sandwiches or can be incorporated into Tempting Turkey Pot Pie, p. 152!

1/4 tsp onion powder
1/4 tsp garlic powder
1/4 tsp coarse ground black pepper
1/4 tsp salt
1 uncooked turkey breast (about 5 lb), thawed
1 Tbsp all-purpose flour
1 roasting bag

1. Preheat oven to 350°F. In a small bowl, combine onion powder, garlic powder, pepper, and salt—set aside.

2. Rinse turkey and pat dry. Loosen skin with knife, then cut skin down one side of turkey breast. Pull skin aside, sprinkle turkey with seasonings, and replace skin.

3. Place flour in roasting bag and shake to coat. Add turkey to roasting bag and close bag using nylon tie that accompanies it. Cut six 1/2-inch slits in top of bag to allow steam to escape. Insert meat thermometer into breast through one of the slits in the bag.

4. Bake approximately 2 hours or until the meat thermometer registers at least 170°F—the meat should be tender and no longer pink. Remove from oven and allow meat to stand 20 minutes before slicing—discard skin.

PREPARATION TIME
15 minutes

BAKING TIME
2 hours

SERVINGS 26

SERVING SIZE
3 oz

EXCHANGES/CHOICES
2 Lean Meat

CALORIES 80
CALORIES FROM FAT 0

TOTAL FAT 0 g
SATURATED FAT <1 g
TRANS FAT 0 g

CHOLESTEROL 50 mg

SODIUM 55 mg

CARBOHYDRATE 0 g
DIETARY FIBER 0 g
SUGARS 0 g

PROTEIN 18 g

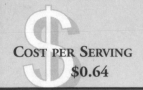
TEMPTING TURKEY POT PIE

PREPARATION TIME
25 minutes

BAKING TIME
30 minutes

SERVINGS 5

SERVING SIZE
1 1/2 cup

EXCHANGES/ CHOICES
3 Starch
1 Vegetable
3 Lean Meat

CALORIES 405
CALORIES FROM FAT 80

TOTAL FAT 9 g
SATURATED FAT 2 g

TRANS FAT <1 g

CHOLESTEROL 60 mg

SODIUM 790 mg

CARBOHYDRATE 49 g
DIETARY FIBER 3 g
SUGARS 10 g

PROTEIN 30 g

Plan to cook Golden Roasted Turkey Breast, p. 151, earlier in the week and use leftovers for this pot pie!

Pot Pie
3 Tbsp light stick margarine
1/3 cup all-purpose flour
1/4 tsp salt
1/8 tsp garlic powder
1/8 tsp ground black pepper
2 cups water
3/4 cup fat-free milk
2 tsp sodium-free instant chicken bouillon granules
1 15-oz can no salt added mixed vegetables, drained
1 small onion (approximately 3 oz), finely diced
2 1/2 cups shredded turkey breast
Cooking spray

Topping
2 cups all purpose reduced-fat baking mix
2/3 cup fat-free milk

1. Preheat oven to 400°F. Melt margarine in a large saucepan over medium heat. Stir in flour, salt, garlic powder, and pepper—a thick paste will form. Add water, milk, and bouillon—stir with a wire whisk until mixture thickens slightly.

2. Add mixed vegetables, onion, and turkey. Stir to combine. Spoon into a 2-quart casserole coated with cooking spray and set aside.

3. Place all-purpose baking mix and milk in a mixing bowl, then stir to combine. Drop dough by rounded tablespoons onto top of turkey mixture. 4. Bake uncovered for 30 minutes or until biscuit topping is golden and filling is bubbly.

SPUNKY SPAGHETTI SAUCE

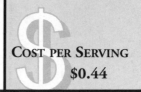

COST PER SERVING
$0.44

Here's a versatile meat sauce that can be served over steaming spaghetti or any hot pasta. It even works in lasagna!

1 lb ground round
1 tsp (or 1 clove) minced garlic
2 Tbsp dried parsley
1 tsp dried basil
1 tsp dried crushed oregano
3/4 tsp salt
4 dashes Red Hot sauce
4 Tbsp Worcestershire sauce
2 15-oz cans tomato Sauce
1 6-oz can no salt added tomato paste
1 14.5-oz can no salt added diced tomatoes

1. In a large skillet, brown ground round over medium-high heat, then drain well.

2. Add remaining ingredients and simmer, covered, for 30 minutes. Stir often.

PREPARATION TIME
40 minutes

SERVINGS 16

SERVING SIZE
1/2 cup

EXCHANGES/CHOICES
1/2 Starch
1 Lean Meat

CALORIES 70
CALORIES FROM FAT 15

TOTAL FAT 2 g
SATURATED FAT <1 g
TRANS FAT 0 g

CHOLESTEROL 15 mg

SODIUM 510 mg

CARBOHYDRATE 8 g
DIETARY FIBER 2 g
SUGARS 4 g

PROTEIN 7 g

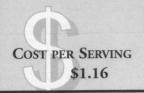

STUFFED PEPPER SLICES

PREPARATION TIME
15 minutes

BAKING TIME
1 hour

CHILLING TIME
2 hours

SERVINGS 6

SERVING SIZE
3 slices

EXCHANGES/CHOICES
1/2 Starch
3 Vegetable
2 Lean Meat

CALORIES 195
CALORIES FROM FAT 40

TOTAL FAT 5 g
SATURATED FAT 2 g
TRANS FAT <1 g

CHOLESTEROL 45 mg

SODIUM 580 mg

CARBOHYDRATE 22 g
DIETARY FIBER 4 g
SUGARS 8 g

PROTEIN 19 g

This unique version of stuffed peppers is a great way to use leftover rice or corn.

6 medium-sized (approximately 5 oz each)
   green peppers
1 lb ground round
1 cup cooked unseasoned brown rice or corn
1 small onion (approximately 3 oz), finely diced
1/4 cup fat-free milk
1/8 tsp ground black pepper
1/4 tsp salt
Cooking spray
1 15-oz can tomato sauce

1. Cut tops from peppers and discard. Remove seeds, then set peppers aside.

2. In a large bowl, combine ground round, rice or corn, onion, milk, pepper, and salt; mix well. Stuff peppers with meat mixture, cover, and refrigerate for at least 2 hours.

3. Preheat oven to 350°F. Remove peppers from the refrigerator and cut each into 3 slices. Arrange overlapping slices in a 9 × 13-inch baking dish coated with cooking spray, and top with tomato sauce.

4. Cover with foil and bake for 45 minutes. Remove foil and continue baking an additional 15 minutes.

Mexican Scramble

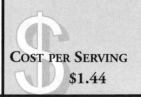
Cost per Serving
$1.44

This simple and spicy stovetop meal is a great way to use a remaining small serving of macaroni or other pasta.

1 lb ground round
1 large onion (approximately 8 oz), chopped
1/2 large green pepper (approximately 3 oz), diced
1 15.25-oz can no salt added corn, drained
1 10-oz can tomatoes and green chilies
1 8-oz can tomato sauce
1/8 tsp ground black pepper
1 tsp to 1 Tbsp chili powder, according to taste
1 cup cooked macaroni (or any small pasta) cooked
   without oil or salt
1 Tbsp cornstarch dissolved in
1/4 cup cold water

1. In a large skillet over medium heat, brown and drain ground round.

2. Add onion, green pepper, corn, tomatoes and green chilies, tomato sauce, pepper, and chili powder; mix well. Cook uncovered over medium heat for 15 minutes; stir periodically.

3. Add macaroni and cornstarch dissolved in water; stir well. Continue cooking and stirring over medium heat until mixture thickens, about 2 to 3 minutes.

Preparation Time
35 minutes

Servings 4

Serving Size
1 1/2 cups

Exchanges/Choices
1 1/2 Starch
3 Vegetable
3 Lean Meat

Calories 325
Calories from Fat 65

Total Fat 7 g
Saturated Fat 3 g
Trans Fat <1 g

Cholesterol 70 mg

Sodium 720 mg

Carbohydrate 36 g
Dietary Fiber 6 g
Sugars 14 g

Protein 28 g

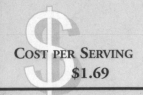

COST PER SERVING
$1.69

BEEF AND BROCCOLI STROGANOFF

PREPARATION TIME
15 minutes

COOKING TIME
35 minutes

SERVINGS 7

SERVING SIZE
3/4 cup meat and
3/4 cup noodles

EXCHANGES/CHOICES
2 Starch
1 Vegetable
3 Lean Meat

CALORIES 345
CALORIES FROM FAT 70

TOTAL FAT 8 g
SATURATED FAT 2 g
TRANS FAT <1 g

CHOLESTEROL 45 mg

SODIUM 345 mg

CARBOHYDRATE 38 g
DIETARY FIBER 4 g
SUGARS 5 g

PROTEIN 25 g

Crisp-tender broccoli adds color and enhances the flavor of traditional beef stroganoff.

1 lb round steak, partially frozen
6 Tbsp all-purpose flour, divided
Cooking spray
1 Tbsp corn oil
1 clove (or 1 tsp) garlic, minced
1 cup fresh sliced mushrooms
1 small onion (approximately 3 oz), finely diced
2 Tbsp light margarine
3/4 tsp salt
1/4 tsp ground black pepper
1 tsp sodium-free beef bouillon granules dissolved in
1 1/2 cups warm water
1 cup fat-free sour cream
2 1/2 cups lightly steamed small broccoli florets
5 cups cooked cholesterol-free egg noodles

1. Remove fat from meat, and slice meat across the grain into bite-sized pieces. Place 3 Tbsp flour in a large zip-top plastic bag. Add meat in two batches and shake to coat.

2. In a large nonstick skillet coated with cooking spray, heat corn oil over medium heat. Add meat and brown. Add garlic, mushrooms, and onion, then cook for 5 minutes. Add margarine and melt.

3. Stir in 2 Tbsp flour until liquid forms a paste. Stir in salt, pepper, and bouillon dissolved in water. Continue cooking 10 minutes, stirring frequently.

4. Stir remaining 1 Tbsp flour into sour cream, then add to meat mixture. Cook for 5 minutes, stirring frequently, but do not boil.

5. Toss in steamed broccoli, spoon over noodles, and serve immediately.

Stovetop Swiss Steak

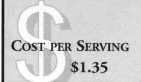
Try mashed potatoes as a tasty accompaniment!

Cooking spray
1 lb round steak, cut into 5 equal portions with fat
  removed
1 8-oz can no salt added tomato sauce
1/3 cup water
1 Tbsp Worcestershire sauce
1/4 cup finely diced onion
1/4 tsp salt
1/8 tsp ground black pepper
1/8 tsp crushed oregano
1 Tbsp dried parsley flakes
1 8.5-oz can no salt added peas, drained and rinsed

1. Warm a large nonstick skillet coated with cooking spray
   over medium-high heat. Add steak and brown on both
   sides. Drain off any fat.

2. In a small bowl, combine tomato sauce, water,
   Worcestershire sauce, onion, salt, pepper, oregano, and
   parsley; mix well. Pour over meat in skillet, cover, and
   simmer for 30 minutes or until meat is tender.

3. Gently stir in peas and cook an additional 2 to 3
   minutes until peas are thoroughly heated.

PREPARATION TIME
10 minutes

COOKING TIME
45 minutes

SERVINGS 5

SERVING SIZE
1/5 recipe

EXCHANGES/CHOICES
1/2 Starch
1 Vegetable
3 Lean Meat

CALORIES 185
CALORIES FROM FAT 40

TOTAL FAT 5 g
SATURATED FAT 1 g
TRANS FAT <1 g

CHOLESTEROL 60 mg

SODIUM 235 mg

CARBOHYDRATE 12 g
DIETARY FIBER 4 g
SUGARS 6 g

PROTEIN 23 g

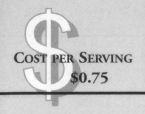

BOUNTIFUL BEEF STEW

PREPARATION TIME
20 minutes

COOKING TIME
1 hour, 10 minutes

SERVINGS 10

SERVING SIZE
1 cup

EXCHANGES/ CHOICES
1/2 Starch
2 Vegetable
1 Lean Meat

CALORIES 125
CALORIES FROM FAT 20

TOTAL FAT 2 g
SATURATED FAT <1 g
TRANS FAT 0 g

CHOLESTEROL 25 mg

SODIUM 535 mg

CARBOHYDRATE 18 g
DIETARY FIBER 2 g
SUGARS 7 g

PROTEIN 9 g

This hearty, filling stew uses one of the least expensive cuts of meat.

1 46-oz can tomato juice
3 cups water
2 tsp sodium-free instant beef bouillon granules
1 lb stew beef, cut into 1-inch cubes, fat trimmed
 (may substitute leftover round steak or beef roast)
1 large onion (approximately 8 oz), coarsely chopped
2 large carrots (approximately 5 oz each), peeled and diced
3 medium potatoes (approximately 5 oz each), peeled and cubed
1/8 tsp ground black pepper
1 Tbsp flour dissolved in 1/4 cup cold water

1. In a 1-gallon pot, combine tomato juice, 3 cups water, bouillon, stew beef, onion, carrots, and potatoes. Cover and bring to a boil over medium-high heat.

2. Decrease heat until stew is at a simmer, and cook for 45 minutes, stirring periodically.

3. Add pepper and flour dissolved in water, stir to combine, then simmer uncovered 15 minutes more.

WESTERN FRITTATA

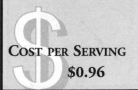
COST PER SERVING
$0.96

A frittata is an Italian omelet in which the "fillings" are combined with the eggs before the eggs are cooked. Any leftover meats or vegetables can be substituted for the ground chuck and vegetables in this recipe.

1/2 lb ground round
1/2 medium onion (approximately 2 1/2 oz), chopped
1/2 green pepper (approximately 2 1/2 oz), diced
1/4 tsp seasoned salt
1/4 tsp ground black pepper
2 Tbsp light margarine
1 2-lb bag frozen shredded hash brown potatoes, thawed
1/4 tsp salt
1 egg + 4 egg whites
1/3 cup fat-free milk
1 cup finely shredded fat-free cheddar cheese

1. In a 12-inch nonstick skillet, brown ground round along with onion and green pepper. Drain well. Stir in seasoned salt and pepper. Remove meat mixture from skillet and set aside. Wipe drippings from skillet.

2. Add margarine to skillet and melt over low heat. Add hash brown potatoes. Sprinkle evenly with salt and toss to coat. Spread potatoes evenly over bottom of skillet. Spread meat mixture evenly over potatoes.

3. In a small bowl, combine egg, egg whites, and milk; whisk well. Pour evenly over ingredients in skillet. Cover and cook over low heat about 20 minutes or until potatoes are tender.

4. Sprinkle evenly with cheese, cover, and cook for an additional 5 minutes or until cheese is melted. Cut into 6 equal wedges and serve immediately.

PREPARATION TIME
45 minutes

SERVINGS 6

SERVING SIZE
2-inch wedge

EXCHANGES/CHOICES
2 Starch
2 Lean Meat
1/2 Fat

CALORIES 285
CALORIES FROM FAT 65

TOTAL FAT 7 g
SATURATED FAT 2 g
TRANS FAT <1 g

CHOLESTEROL 60 mg

SODIUM 495 mg

CARBOHYDRATE 34 g
DIETARY FIBER 2 g
SUGARS 3 g

PROTEIN 21 g

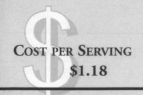

DIJON-CRUSTED BEEF ROAST

PREPARATION TIME
10 minutes

COOKING TIME
2 hours, 30 minutes

STANDING TIME
10 minutes

SERVINGS 13

SERVING SIZE
3 oz

EXCHANGES/ CHOICES
3 Lean Meat

CALORIES 120
CALORIES FROM FAT 25

TOTAL FAT 3 g
SATURATED FAT <1 g
TRANS FAT 0 g

CHOLESTEROL 45 mg

SODIUM 255 mg

CARBOHYDRATE 4 g
DIETARY FIBER 0 g
SUGARS 1 g

PROTEIN 19 g

Dijon mustard and seasoned bread crumbs create a unique crust for this succulent roast.

1 2.5-lb boneless top round roast, fat trimmed
Butter-flavored cooking spray
1/2 tsp ground black pepper
1/2 tsp salt
1/2 cup dry unseasoned bread crumbs
2 Tbsp dried parsley flakes
2 tsp (or 2 cloves) minced garlic
1/4 cup Dijon mustard

1. Preheat oven to 325°F. Place roast in a roasting pan coated with cooking spray and sprinkle evenly with pepper and salt.

2. In a small bowl, combine bread crumbs and parsley.

3. In another small bowl, mix together garlic and mustard. Spread mustard mixture on top and sides of roast.

4. Firmly pat bread crumb mixture onto mustard. Spray top and sides of roast with cooking spray. Insert meat thermometer into center of roast. Cover with foil and bake for 2 hours.

5. Remove foil and continue baking for an additional 30 minutes or until crust is lightly browned, the meat thermometer registers 170°F, and meat is no longer pink in the center.

6. Remove from oven and let stand 20 minutes before slicing.

Eggs in a Basket

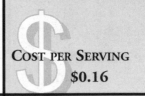
Lightly toast the leftover bread circles, then sprinkle them with cinnamon or top them with 100% fruit spread.

Butter-flavored cooking spray
4 slices whole-wheat bread
4 medium eggs
4 dashes salt
4 dashes ground black pepper

1. Coat a large nonstick skillet and both sides of the bread slices with cooking spray. Place the bread in skillet, invert a 2-inch glass over the center of each slice, and cut out a circle. Set circles aside. Heat bread slices over medium-low heat.

2. Break 1 egg into center of each bread slice, and sprinkle with a dash of salt and a dash of pepper. Cook until egg white begins to turn white (about 3 minutes). Turn bread/egg with spatula and continue cooking until egg yolk is firm (about 3 more minutes).

Preparation Time
10 minutes

Servings 4

Serving Size
1 egg in a basket

Exchanges/Changes
1/2 Starch
1 Med Fat Meat

Calories 110
Calories from Fat 55

Total Fat 6 g
Saturated Fat 1 g
Trans Fat 0 g

Cholesterol 210 mg

Sodium 145 mg

Carbohydrate 7 g
Dietary Fiber 1 g
Sugars 1 g

Protein 8 g

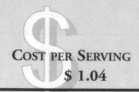

HAWAIIAN QUESADILLAS

PREPARATION TIME
10 minutes

COOKING TIME
4 minutes

SERVINGS 4

SERVING SIZE
1 quesadilla

EXCHANGES/CHOICES
3 1/2 Starch
1 1/2 Fat

CALORIES 476
CALORIES FROM FAT 72

TOTAL FAT 8 g
SATURATED FAT 1 g
TRANS FAT 0 g

CHOLESTEROL 19 mg

SODIUM 1,800 mg

CARBOHYDRATE 71 g
DIETARY FIBER 5 g
SUGARS 23 g

PROTEIN 25 g

A quick and delicious variation on a traditional Mexican favorite. Barbecue sauce blends wonderfully with ham and pineapple!

1/2 cup honey barbecue sauce
8 7-inch whole-wheat soft flour tortillas
4 oz diced cooked ham
1/2 cup diced red onion
1/2 cup diced green pepper
1/8 tsp garlic powder
1 8-oz can pineapple tidbits, packed in juice, drained
1 cup fat-free shredded mozzarella cheese

1. Spread 2 Tbsp of barbecue sauce on one tortilla.

2. Top the tortilla with 1 oz ham, 2 Tbsp red onion, 2 Tbsp green pepper, light sprinkle of garlic powder, 1/4 cup pineapple, and 1/4 cup cheese.

3. Cover with a second tortilla. Microwave for 60 seconds. Let tortilla set for 1 minute, then use a pizza cutter to divide each tortilla into four sections.

GRILLED ASIAN PORK KABOBS

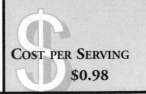
Kabobs can be assembled ahead and refrigerated until cooking time. Serve grilled kabobs with hot brown rice.

Sauce
2 Tbsp reduced-sodium soy sauce
1/4 cup ketchup
2 Tbsp packed brown sugar
1/4 tsp garlic powder
2 Tbsp cold water

Kabobs
4 8-inch bamboo skewers, soaked in water for 30 minutes
8 oz. raw lean pork, cut into eight 1 1/2-inch cubes
4 pineapple rings canned in juice, each cut into 4
   equal-size pieces
1 small red onion (approximately 3 oz), cut into 4 pieces
4 cherry tomatoes (or 1 small tomato cut into 4 pieces)
4 mushrooms

1. Preheat grill to medium heat.

2. In a small bowl, whisk together sauce ingredients. Set aside.

3. Push onto each skewer in the following order: 1 pork cube, 4 slices pineapple, 1/4 onion, 1 pork cube, 1 tomato, and 1 mushroom.

4. Brush kabobs with half of sauce.

5. Grill covered over medium heat for 15–20 minutes, or until pork is cooked through and no longer pink (turn kabobs to allow for even cooking); baste with remaining sauce halfway through.

PREPARATION TIME
20 minutes

GRILLING TIME
15–20 minutes

SERVINGS 4

SERVING SIZE
1 kabob

EXCHANGES/CHOICES
1 1/2 Carbohydrate
1 Lean Meat

CALORIES 147
CALORIES FROM FAT 16

TOTAL FAT 2 g
SATURATED FAT <1 g
TRANS FAT 0 g

CHOLESTEROL 30 mg

SODIUM 491 mg

CARBOHYDRATE 21 g
DIETARY FIBER 1 g
SUGARS 16 g

PROTEIN 13 g

SEASONED PAN-FRIED CATFISH

Instant potato flakes lend a crunchy coating to the tender catfish fillets.

1/2 cup instant potato flakes
1/2 tsp seasoned salt
1/8 tsp ground black pepper
12 oz boneless, skinless catfish fillets
1 medium egg, beaten
Butter-flavored cooking spray

1. In a shallow dish, combine potato flakes, seasoned salt, and pepper. Dip catfish fillets in beaten egg, then coat well with seasoned potato mixture.

2. Place in a large nonstick skillet coated generously with cooking spray, and cook over medium heat until fillets are golden, about 8–10 minutes.

3. Spray remaining uncooked side of fillets with cooking spray, turn over, and continue cooking until golden and fish flakes easily with a fork (about 8–10 more minutes). Turn only once during cooking.

FANTASTIC FISH TACOS

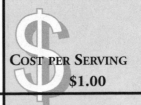
COST PER SERVING
$1.00

Marinated fish brings a unique taste to these soft tacos, while shredded cabbage adds crunch.

8 oz boneless, skinless white fish filets (i.e., orange roughy)
2 Tbsp fresh-squeezed lime juice
1/8 tsp black pepper
1/4 tsp salt
1/4 tsp chili powder
1/4 tsp paprika
Cooking spray
4 8-inch whole-wheat flour tortillas
1/2 avocado, mashed
1/4 cup finely shredded low-fat cheddar cheese
1/3 cup salsa
3/4 cup shredded cabbage
2 Tbsp fat-free sour cream
Hot sauce (optional)

1. Place fish in a shallow dish and sprinkle evenly with lime juice, black pepper, salt, chili powder, and paprika. Cover and chill 30–60 minutes to marinate.

2. Preheat oven to 375°F.

3. Coat a large piece of foil with cooking spray. Place fish on the foil in a single layer. Seal foil and bake packet for 8–10 minutes, or until fish flakes easily with a fork.

4. Heat tortillas in microwave for 20–30 seconds (or wrapped in foil in oven for 2–3 minutes).

5. Spread each tortilla with avocado, then layer with fish, cheese, salsa, cabbage, and sour cream. Fold each tortilla in half.

PREPARATION TIME
20 minutes

MARINATING TIME
30–60 minutes

COOKING TIME
8–10 minutes

SERVINGS 4

SERVING SIZE
1 taco

EXCHANGES/ CHOICES
2 Starch
2 Lean Meat

CALORIES 273
CALORIES FROM FAT 79

TOTAL FAT 9 g
SATURATED FAT 2 g
TRANS FAT 0 g

CHOLESTEROL 41 mg

SODIUM 764 mg

CARBOHYDRATE 31 g
DIETARY FIBER 4 g
SUGARS 3 g

PROTEIN 17 g

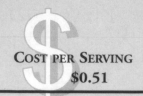

COST PER SERVING
$0.51

TUNA ROLL-UPS

PREPARATION TIME
10 minutes

SERVINGS 2

SERVING SIZE
4 pieces

EXCHANGES/CHOICES
1 Starch
1 Lean Meat
1/2 Fat

CALORIES 127
CALORIES FROM FAT 33

TOTAL FAT 4 g
SATURATED FAT 1 g
TRANS FAT 0 g

CHOLESTEROL 14 mg

SODIUM 305 mg

CARBOHYDRATE 12 g
DIETARY FIBER 2 g
SUGARS 2 g

PROTEIN 12 g

These tasty roll-ups are reminiscent of sushi without the rice. They are best if eaten within a few hours after preparation.

1 3-oz can tuna packed in water
1 Tbsp reduced-fat mayonnaise (or horseradish
    mayonnaise or light wasabi)
1 tsp fresh-squeezed lemon juice
Black pepper to taste
2 slices soft whole-wheat bread
2 Tbsp shredded carrot
2 cucumber spears (4–5 inches in length)

1. Drain tuna and flake with a fork. Stir in mayonnaise, lemon juice, and pepper; mix well.

2. Trim crusts from bread and flatten bread to about 1/16 inch using a rolling pin. Spoon one-half of the tuna mixture down the center of each slice of bread.

3. Sprinkle with carrot and top with a cucumber spear.

4. Roll the bread up tightly around the cucumber spear to enclose the filling. Cut each roll crosswise into 4 pieces and place cut-side up on a serving plate.

Gourmet Grilled Cheese

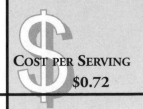
Cost per Serving
$0.72

Here's a calcium boost for those who aren't "milk-drinkers"

2 Tbsp light tub margarine, room temperature
4 slices whole-wheat bread
Cooking spray
4 large tomato slices (approximately 5 oz)
2 slices fat-free processed American cheese
12 thin, large zucchini slices (approximately 3 oz)
1/8 tsp salt-free seasoning blend
Ground black pepper

1. Spread the 2 Tbsp margarine on the four slices of bread. Place 2 slices bread, margarine-side down, in a nonstick skillet coated with cooking spray over medium heat. Top each of these with 2 slices tomato, 1 slice cheese, and 6 slices zucchini.

2. Sprinkle with salt-free seasoning and pepper. Top with the remaining slices of bread, margarine side up.

3. When the sandwiches are lightly browned on one side, turn them over using a spatula. Continue cooking until lightly browned on second side and cheese is melted.

4. Cut each sandwich in half and serve.

Preparation Time
20 minutes

Servings 2

Serving Size
1 sandwich

Exchanges/Choices
1 1/2 Starch
1 Vegetable
1 Lean Meat
1 Fat

Calories 235
Calories from Fat 70

Total Fat 8 g
Saturated Fat 2 g
Trans Fat <1 g

Cholesterol 5 mg

Sodium 665 mg

Carbohydrate 32 g
Dietary Fiber 5 g
Sugars 6 g

Protein 12 g

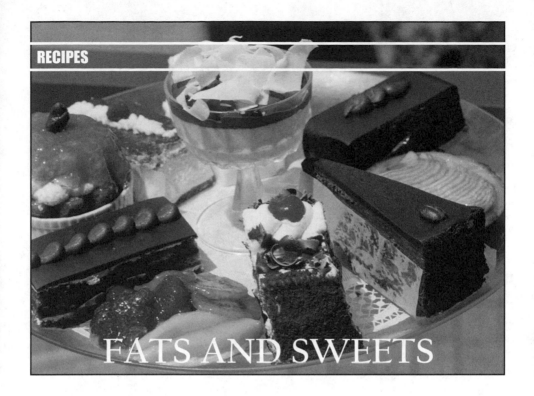

FATS AND SWEETS

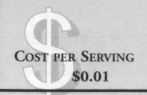

COST PER SERVING
$0.01

HERBED MARGARINE

PREPARATION TIME
5 minutes

CHILLING TIME
1 hour

SERVINGS 48

SERVING SIZE
1 tsp

EXCHANGES/CHOICES
1 Free Food

CALORIES 15
CALORIES FROM FAT 15

TOTAL FAT 2 g
SATURATED FAT <1 g
TRANS FAT 0 g

CHOLESTEROL 0 mg

SODIUM 35 mg

CARBOHYDRATE 0 g
DIETARY FIBER 0 g
SUGARS 0 g

PROTEIN 0 g

Lightly flavored with thyme and dill weed, this spread is marvelous on warm, crusty bread or steaming hot baked potatoes.

2 (8 oz) light tub margarine, softened
1 tsp dried thyme
1 tsp dried dill weed
1/8 tsp salt

1. Place softened margarine in a mixing bowl and stir in thyme, dill weed, and salt.

2. Store in refrigerator in tightly covered container. The spread is best if refrigerated for at least one hour before serving to allow flavors to blend.

VERSATILE VINAIGRETTE

COST PER SERVING
$ 0.24

Drizzle over salad greens, steamed asparagus, or green beans. Even use as a flavorful meat marinade.

1/2 cup red wine vinegar
1/4 cup balsamic vinegar
2 tsp cornstarch
1/4 cup cold water
1/4 tsp dried basil
1/4 tsp dried oregano
1/8 tsp salt
1/8 tsp black pepper
2 tsp (or 2 cloves) minced garlic
2 Tbsp olive oil

1. In a small saucepan, whisk together red wine vinegar, balsamic vinegar, and cornstarch until cornstarch is dissolved.

2. Cook over medium-high heat, whisking frequently until mixture thickens slightly (approximately 3 minutes). Remove pan from heat.

3. Whisk in remaining ingredients. Chill at least 1 hour to allow flavors to blend. Whisk or shake mixture well before serving.

PREPARATION TIME
10 minutes

CHILLING TIME
1 hour

SERVINGS 8

SERVING SIZE
2 Tbsp

EXCHANGES/CHOICES
1 Fat

CALORIES 41
CALORIES FROM FAT 30

TOTAL FAT 3 g
SATURATED FAT <1 g
TRANS FAT 0 g

CHOLESTEROL 0 mg

SODIUM 39 mg

CARBOHYDRATE 3 g
DIETARY FIBER 0 g
SUGARS 2 g

PROTEIN 0 g

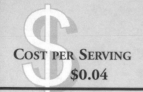

Cost per Serving
$0.04

BASIC BROWN GRAVY

PREPARATION TIME
5 minutes

COOKING TIME
8–10 minutes

SERVINGS 18

SERVING SIZE
2 Tbsp

EXCHANGES/ CHOICES
1/2 Fat

CALORIES 25
CALORIES FROM FAT 10

TOTAL FAT 1 g
SATURATED FAT <1 g
TRANS FAT 0 g

CHOLESTEROL 0 mg

SODIUM 90 mg

CARBOHYDRATE 3 g
DIETARY FIBER 0 g
SUGARS 1 g

PROTEIN 1 g

Serve over biscuits, beef roast, or pork roast.

1 1/2 Tbsp corn oil
1/4 cup all-purpose flour
2 cups fat-free milk
1/2 cup cold water
1/8 tsp ground black pepper
1/8 tsp salt
2 cubes reduced-sodium beef bouillon dissolved in
1/4 cup hot water
Kitchen Bouquet (optional); usually found in spice aisle.

1. Place corn oil in a large skillet over medium-high heat. Combine flour, milk, 1/2 cup cold water, pepper, and salt in a jar, cover tightly, and shake to mix well. Pour milk mixture into hot oil and cook, stirring constantly with a wire whisk, until it begins to thicken, about 1 or 2 minutes.

2. Add bouillon dissolved in hot water and continue cooking, whisking constantly, until thickened, about 3 minutes. If darker brown gravy is preferred, add several drops Kitchen Bouquet until desired color is achieved.

BROILED PINEAPPLE RINGS

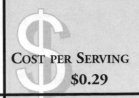

This eye-pleasing dessert is simple and quick. Serve it hot from the oven.

1 20-oz can sliced pineapple rings in juice, drained (1 can should contain 10 rings)
10 maraschino cherries, drained and rinsed
3 Tbsp + 1 tsp light brown sugar
5 tsp light stick margarine, melted
Ground cinnamon

1. Preheat broiler. Lay drained pineapple rings in a single layer on a 9 × 13-inch pan with sides—allow edges of pineapple rings to touch.

2. Place a cherry in the center of each pineapple ring. Sprinkle each pineapple ring with 1 tsp brown sugar, then drizzle with 1/2 tsp margarine. Sprinkle with cinnamon.

3. Place 5 inches from broiler and broil (with oven door cracked) for 5 minutes or until topping is bubbly.

PREPARATION TIME
5 minutes

BROILING TIME
5 minutes

SERVINGS 5

SERVING SIZE
2 slices

EXCHANGES/ CHOICES
1 1/2 Carbohydrate
1/2 Fat

CALORIES 135
CALORIES FROM FAT 35

TOTAL FAT 4 g
SATURATED FAT 1 g
TRANS FAT 0 g

CHOLESTEROL 0 mg

SODIUM 40 mg

CARBOHYDRATE 25 g
DIETARY FIBER 1 g
SUGARS 24 g

PROTEIN 0 g

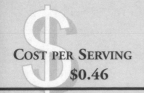

COST PER SERVING
$0.46

CHEERY BLACK CHERRY SALAD

PREPARATION TIME
15 minutes

CHILLING TIME
2 hours

SERVINGS 9

SERVING SIZE
1 square

EXCHANGES/CHOICES
1/2 Fruit
1 Carbohydrate

CALORIES 105
CALORIES FROM FAT 0

TOTAL FAT 0 g
SATURATED FAT 0 g
TRANS FAT 0 g

CHOLESTEROL 5 mg

SODIUM 190 mg

CARBOHYDRATE 19 g
DIETARY FIBER 1 g
SUGARS 11 g

PROTEIN 4 g

Serve on a lettuce leaf and garnish with lightly toasted coconut if desired.

1 15-oz can pitted dark sweet cherries
1 8-oz package reduced-fat cream cheese, softened
1 tsp vanilla extract
1 8-oz container frozen fat-free whipped topping, thawed
1 8-oz can crushed pineapple in juice, drained

1. Drain juice off cherries and reserve. Slice cherries in half.

2. In a large bowl, whip softened cream cheese with an electric mixer until light and fluffy. Add vanilla extract, 5 Tbsp reserved cherry juice, and whipped topping. Whip until combined.

3. Stir in cherries and drained pineapple. Spoon into a 9 × 9-inch serving dish and chill for 2 hours. Cut into 3 × 3-inch squares before serving (it will be very soft, so you may prefer to spoon it out).

CREAMY FRUIT WHIP

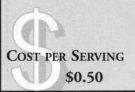

For a special touch, garnish each dish with a whole strawberry or a sprinkle of fresh blueberries.

2 8-oz packages fat-free cream cheese
1 tub sugar-free lemonade mix (enough to make 2 quarts lemonade)
1 8-oz container frozen fat-free whipped topping, thawed
1 cup crushed strawberries (fresh or unsweetened frozen; approximately 24 medium berries)

1. Place cream cheese and lemonade mix in large bowl. Beat with an electric mixer on medium speed until fluffy and smooth. Gently fold in whipped topping, then strawberries, mixing until combined.

2. Pour into individual serving dishes if desired. Cover and refrigerate 2 hours or until of a slightly firmer consistency. Stir twice during chilling if not in individual dishes.

PREPARATION TIME
15 minutes

CHILLING TIME
2 hours

SERVINGS 10

SERVING SIZE
1/2 cup

EXCHANGES/CHOICES
1 Carbohydrate

CALORIES 100
CALORIES FROM FAT 0

TOTAL FAT 0 g
SATURATED FAT 0 g
TRANS FAT 0 g

CHOLESTEROL 5 mg

SODIUM 360 mg

CARBOHYDRATE 14 g
DIETARY FIBER 1 g
SUGARS 6 g

PROTEIN 7 g

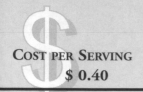

RAINBOW PARFAITS

PREPARATION TIME
10 minutes

SERVINGS 4

SERVING SIZE
1 parfait

EXCHANGES/CHOICES
3 Carbohydrate

CALORIES 195
CALORIES FROM FAT 20

TOTAL FAT 2 g
SATURATED FAT 1 g
TRANS FAT 0 g

CHOLESTEROL 0 mg

SODIUM 70 mg

CARBOHYDRATE 42 g
DIETARY FIBER 3 g
SUGARS 33 g

PROTEIN 2 g

Here's a refreshing and very simple dessert!

2 cups rainbow sherbet
1 6-oz container no sugar added, fat-free vanilla yogurt
1/4 cup raspberry 100% fruit spread, heated

1. Place 1/2 cup sherbet in each of four parfait glasses.

2. Drizzle each with 1/2 container yogurt, then 1 Tbsp
   heated raspberry spread. Serve immediately.

Chocolate Lovers' Frozen Mousse

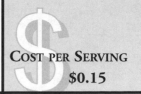
This creamy chocolate mousse is laced with mini chocolate chips.

2 1.4-oz boxes sugar-free, fat-free instant chocolate
   pudding mix
3 cups fat-free milk
1/4 tsp cinnamon
16 oz frozen fat-free whipped topping, thawed
1/2 cup mini chocolate chips

1. Place pudding mix, milk, and cinnamon in a large mixing
   bowl. Beat with an electric mixer on medium speed until
   pudding mix is dissolved.

2. Add whipped topping and mix on low speed until
   smooth. Gently stir in chocolate chips.

3. Cover tightly and freeze until firm (about 3 hours). To
   serve, scoop into bowls using an ice cream scoop.

Preparation Time
10 minutes

Freezing Time
3 hours

Servings 24

Serving Size
1/2 cup

Exchanges/Choices
1 Carbohydrate

Calories 70
Calories from Fat 10

Total Fat 1 g
Saturated Fat <1 g
Trans Fat 0 g

Cholesterol 0 mg

Sodium 130 mg

Carbohydrate 13 g
Dietary Fiber 0 g
Sugars 6 g

Protein 2 g

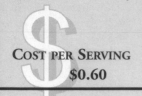

Cost per Serving
$0.60

Banana-Split Parfaits

Preparation Time
20 minutes

Servings 4

Serving Size
1 parfait

Exchanges/Choices
2 1/2 Carbohydrate

Calories 185
Calories from Fat 5

Total Fat 1 g
Saturated Fat <1 g
Trans Fat 0 g

Cholesterol 0 mg

Sodium 380 mg

Carbohydrate 39 g
Dietary Fiber 2 g
Sugars 25 g

Protein 6 g

These parfaits are reminiscent of the old-fashioned favorite banana split.

1 1.4-oz box sugar-free, fat-free instant chocolate pudding mix
2 cups fat-free milk
1 medium banana (approximately 5 oz), sliced
1 8-oz can crushed pineapple in juice, drained
1/4 cup strawberry 100% fruit spread
1/4 cup frozen "lite" whipped topping, thawed
4 maraschino cherries

1. In a mixing bowl, combine pudding and milk, then beat with an electric mixer on low speed until well blended (about 1 to 2 minutes).

2. Layer 1/4 cup pudding in each of 4 parfait glasses. Let stand 5 minutes, then top each with 1/4 of banana slices, 1/4 of pineapple, 1 Tbsp strawberry fruit spread, and another 1/4 cup pudding.

3. Garnish with 1 Tbsp whipped topping and a maraschino cherry. Serve immediately.

Rich Chocolate Fudge Cake

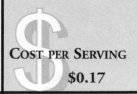
While this cake bakes, a layer of rich chocolate sauce appears on the bottom. Tastes great served with a dollop of lite whipped topping or vanilla ice milk.

1 cup all-purpose reduced-fat baking mix
1/2 cup Splenda sugar blend for baking
3 Tbsp plus 1/3 cup unsweetened cocoa powder
Cooking spray
1/2 cup fat-free milk
1 teaspoon vanilla
1 2/3 cup hot tap water

1. Preheat oven to 350°F.

2. Mix baking mix, 1/4 cup Splenda, and 3 Tbsp cocoa in a 9 × 9-inch baking dish coated with cooking spray.

3. Stir in milk and vanilla until well blended.

4. Sprinkle evenly with remaining 1/3 cup cocoa and 1/4 cup Splenda. Pour on water.

5. Bake 40 minutes or until top is firm.

6. Portion into nine 3 × 3-inch squares. Serve at once in dessert bowls with sauce spooned over cake.

Preparation Time
15 minutes

Baking Time
40 minutes

Servings 9

Serving Size
1 square or 1/9 recipe

Exchanges/Choices
1 1/2 Carbohydrate

Calories 117
Calories from Fat 22

Total Fat 2 g
Saturated Fat 1 g
Trans Fat <1 g

Cholesterol 0 mg

Sodium 183 mg

Carbohydrate 23 g
Dietary Fiber 2 g
Sugars 12 g

Protein 3 g

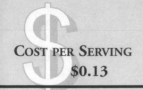

Cost per Serving
$0.13

Pumpkin Bars

Preparation Time
10 minutes

Baking Time
30–40 minutes

Servings 24

Serving Size
1 square

Exchanges/Choices
1 Carbohydrate

Calories 85
Calories from Fat 5

Total Fat 1 g
Saturated Fat <1 g
Trans Fat 0 g

Cholesterol 18 mg

Sodium 42 mg

Carbohydrate 19 g
Dietary Fiber 1 g
Sugars 14 g

Protein 1 g

A fall favorite that's a year-round treat!

Cake
Cooking spray
Flour for dusting pan
1/2 cup whole-wheat flour
1/2 cup white flour
1 tsp cinnamon
1/2 tsp baking powder
1/2 tsp baking soda
2 medium eggs (or 1/2 cup liquid egg substitute)
1/2 cup unsweetened applesauce
1 cup Splenda sugar blend for baking
1 cup solid pack pumpkin puree
3/4 cup raisins

Glaze
1/2 cup sifted confectioners' sugar
1 Tbsp sugar-free maple-flavored syrup

1. Preheat oven to 350°F. Coat a 9 × 13-inch baking pan with cooking spray and dust with flour.

2. In a medium bowl, stir together flours, cinnamon, baking powder, and baking soda; set aside. In a large bowl stir the eggs, applesauce, and Splenda until smooth. Stir in the pumpkin, then the dry ingredients. Finally, add the raisins.

3. Pour the mixture into the prepared baking pan and spread evenly. Bake for 30–40 minutes. Allow bars to cool before adding glaze.

4. To make the glaze, stir together the confectioners' sugar with the syrup. If the glaze is too thick to drizzle from a spoon, just add a bit of water.

5. Drizzle over the cooled pumpkin bars before cutting into 2 × 2-inch squares.

Chocolate Peanut Butter Drops

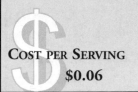
Cost per Serving
$0.06

So simple! Ricotta cheese is the secret ingredient in these fudgy treats.

2 Tbsp light stick margarine
1/3 cup plain or chunky peanut butter
1 oz square unsweetened chocolate
1/3 cup part skim ricotta cheese
1/2 cup Splenda granular
1 tsp vanilla extract
Powdered sugar (optional)

1. Melt margarine, peanut butter, and chocolate for 60 seconds in microwave.

2. Cool slightly, then add ricotta, sweetener, and vanilla. Blend completely with an electric mixer.

3. Drop by teaspoonfuls onto wax paper. Refrigerate for 1 hour prior to serving, then dust with powdered sugar if desired. Store in refrigerator.

Preparation Time
15 minutes

Chilling Time
1 hour

Servings 24

Serving Size
1 drop

Exchanges/Choices
1 Fat

Calories 38
Calories from Fat 28

Total Fat 3 g
Saturated Fat 1 g
Trans Fat 0 g

Cholesterol 1 mg

Sodium 28 mg

Carbohydrate 2 g
Dietary Fiber 0 g
Sugars 1 g

Protein 1 g

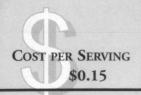

COST PER SERVING
$0.15

PEACH COBBLE-UP

PREPARATION TIME
15 minutes

BAKING TIME
30 minutes

SERVINGS 9

SERVING SIZE
1 square

EXCHANGES/CHOICES
1 1/2 Carbohydrate

CALORIES 105
CALORIES FROM FAT 20

TOTAL FAT 2 g
SATURATED FAT <1 g
TRANS FAT <1 g

CHOLESTEROL 0 mg

SODIUM 165 mg

CARBOHYDRATE 21 g
DIETARY FIBER 1 g
SUGARS 12 g

PROTEIN 2 g

Serve warm with a steaming cup of coffee or tea!

1 cup all-purpose reduced-fat baking mix
1/4 cup packed dark brown sugar
1/4 tsp ground nutmeg
1 tsp ground cinnamon
1 Tbsp light stick margarine, softened
1/3 cup fat-free milk
Cooking spray
1 15-oz can sliced peaches in juice, drained and with juice reserved

1. Preheat oven to 400°F. In a large mixing bowl, combine biscuit baking mix, brown sugar, nutmeg, and cinnamon. Using an electric mixer on low, mix in softened margarine until mixture is crumbly. Add milk and blend thoroughly.

2. Spread batter evenly on the bottom of a 9 × 9- inch square pan coated with cooking spray. Place peach slices on top of batter. Pour reserved juice evenly over peaches.

3. Bake for 30 minutes. Slice into 3 × 3-inch squares. Refrigerate leftovers, then reheat before serving.

CLASSIC APPLE CRISP

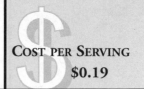

COST PER SERVING
$0.19

If you have apples that have lost their crispness, don't throw them away-use them in this cobbler!

Fruit
3 cups thinly sliced, peeled apples
Cooking spray
1 Tbsp lemon juice
1/2 tsp ground cinnamon
1/4 cup sugar

Topping
1/4 cup all-purpose flour
1/2 cup brown sugar
2 Tbsp light stick margarine
1/4 cup quick-cooking oats

1. Preheat oven to 375°F. Place apples in a 9 × 9-inch square baking dish coated with cooking spray. Sprinkle with lemon juice, cinnamon, and sugar. Cover with foil and bake for 45 minutes.

2. In a mixing bowl, combine flour, brown sugar, and margarine using a pastry blender and mixing until crumbly. Stir in oats.

3. Remove foil from cooked fruit and top with oatmeal mixture. Bake uncovered for 20 minutes or until topping is golden. Portion into nine 3 × 3-inch squares.

PREPARATION TIME
30 minutes

BAKING TIME
1 hour, 5 minutes

SERVINGS 9

SERVING SIZE
1 square

EXCHANGES/CHOICES
2 Carbohydrate

CALORIES 130
CALORIES FROM FAT 20

TOTAL FAT 3 g
SATURATED FAT <1 g
TRANS FAT <1 g

CHOLESTEROL 0 mg

SODIUM 30 mg

CARBOHYDRATE 28 g
DIETARY FIBER 1 g
SUGARS 23 g

PROTEIN 1 g

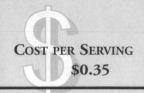

SIMPLE STRAWBERRY SHORTCAKE

PREPARATION TIME
25 minutes

BAKING TIME
10–14 minutes

SERVINGS 10

SERVING SIZE
1 shortcake

EXCHANGES/CHOICES
3 Carbohydrate
1/2 Fat

CALORIES 225
CALORIES FROM FAT 45

TOTAL FAT 5 g
SATURATED FAT 1 g
TRANS FAT <1 g

CHOLESTEROL 0 mg

SODIUM 350 mg

CARBOHYDRATE 44 g
DIETARY FIBER 1 g
SUGARS 22 g

PROTEIN 3 g

Warmed strawberry fruit spread serves as a quick topping for these simple shortcakes.

Shortcakes
2 1/3 cups all-purpose reduced-fat baking mix
2 Tbsp sugar
3 Tbsp light stick margarine, melted
1/2 cup fat-free milk
1/2 tsp vanilla extract

Topping
1 1/4 cups strawberry 100% fruit spread, heated
10 Tbsp frozen "lite" whipped topping, thawed

1. Preheat oven to 425°F. Combine baking mix, sugar, margarine, milk, and extract in a large mixing bowl. Stir until ingredients are combined and a soft dough forms—dough will be sticky.

2. Turn dough out onto waxed paper dusted with flour and knead 10 times with floured hands. Using a floured rolling pin, roll dough to 1/2-inch thickness, and cut into 10 cakes with a 2 1/2-inch floured round cookie or biscuit cutter.

3. Place dough on ungreased baking sheet and bake at 425°F for 10–14 minutes or until light golden.

4. Split each warm shortcake in half. Drizzle each bottom with 1 Tbsp heated fruit spread, then top with 1 Tbsp whipped topping. Replace shortcake tops and drizzle each with 1 Tbsp heated fruit spread. Serve immediately.

CINNAMON COFFEECAKE

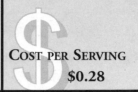
Enjoy at breakfast or as a dessert with fresh fruit on top.

Cake
Cooking spray
2 cups all-purpose flour
1/4 tsp allspice
1 tsp ground cinnamon
1 tsp baking soda
1 tsp baking powder
1/2 cup liquid egg substitute (or 4 egg whites)
2 Tbsp corn oil
1 tsp vanilla extract
1 1/2 cups fat-free sour cream
1/3 cup Splenda sugar blend for baking
1/4 cup packed Splenda brown sugar blend

Topping
1/3 cup all-purpose flour
1/2 cup instant oats
1/4 cup packed Splenda brown sugar blend
1 tsp ground cinnamon
2 Tbsp corn oil stick margarine

1. Preheat oven to 350°F. Coat a 9 × 13-inch pan with cooking spray. Combine flour, cinnamon, allspice, baking soda, and baking powder; mix.

2. In a separate bowl, whisk egg substitute, corn oil, vanilla extract, sour cream, and both Splenda sugar blends.

3. Quickly stir the flour mixture into the sour cream mixture until just thoroughly moistened.

4. Spread the batter into the prepared pan; set aside.

5. In a third bowl, prepare the topping by combining the remaining flour, oats, Splenda brown sugar, corn oil, and cinnamon; mix. Cut margarine in using a fork. Sprinkle the topping over the batter.

6. Bake approximately 25 minutes, or until a toothpick inserted into the cake comes out clean.

PREPARATION TIME
25 minutes

BAKING TIME
25 minutes

SERVINGS 12

SERVING SIZE
1/12 of cake

EXCHANGES/CHOICES
2 1/2 Carbohydrate
1 Fat

CALORIES 230
CALORIES FROM FAT 41

TOTAL FAT 5 g
SATURATED FAT <1 g
TRANS FAT <1 g

CHOLESTEROL 3 mg

SODIUM 192 mg

CARBOHYDRATE 36 g
DIETARY FIBER 1 g
SUGARS 15 g

PROTEIN 6 g

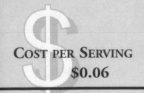

COST PER SERVING
$0.06

VANILLA CUSTARD SAUCE

PREPARATION TIME
10 minutes

BAKING TIME
15 minutes

SERVINGS 19

SERVING SIZE
2 Tbsp

EXCHANGES/CHOICES
1/2 Carbohydrate

CALORIES 25
CALORIES FROM FAT 10

TOTAL FAT 1 g
SATURATED FAT <1 g
TRANS FAT <1 g

CHOLESTEROL 0 mg

SODIUM 35 mg

CARBOHYDRATE 3 g
DIETARY FIBER 0 g
SUGARS 2 g

PROTEIN 2 g

Drizzle over fresh fruit, angel food cake, or leftover muffins that are split in half.

2 cups fat-free milk
2 Tbsp cornstarch
1/2 cup liquid egg substitute
2 Tbsp light stick margarine
1 1/2 tsp vanilla extract
10 packets Aspartame artificial sweetener

1. In a large saucepan, combine milk, cornstarch, and egg substitute. Whisk until well mixed. Add margarine, then place pan over medium heat. Cook uncovered about 8 minutes or until custard thickens. Once custard begins to heat and thicken, whisk constantly to prevent sticking.

2. Remove from heat and whisk in vanilla extract and sweetener. Serve warm.

3. Refrigerate leftovers—will thicken upon chilling. May be eaten cold as custard rather than as a sauce.

BANANA-CREAM FRUIT DIP

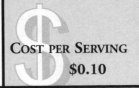

COST PER SERVING
$0.10

Try this simple dip with fresh fruit.

1 0.9-oz package sugar-free, fat-free instant banana-cream
   pudding mix
3/4 cup fat-free milk
1 8-oz can crushed pineapple in juice, drained and with
   juice reserved
1/2 cup fat-free sour cream

1. In a large bowl, combine pudding mix, milk, and
   reserved pineapple juice. Mix with an electric mixer
   until smooth (will be thick). Add sour cream and mix
   again until smooth.

2. Stir in pineapple and chill for 30 minutes.

PREPARATION TIME
10 minutes

CHILLING TIME
30 minutes

SERVINGS 16

SERVING SIZE
2 Tbsp

EXCHANGES/ CHOICES
1/2 Carbohydrate

CALORIES 25
CALORIES FROM FAT 0

TOTAL FAT 0 g
SATURATED FAT 0 g
TRANS FAT 0 g

CHOLESTEROL 0 mg

SODIUM 90 mg

CARBOHYDRATE 4 g
DIETARY FIBER 0 g
SUGARS 2 g

PROTEIN 1 g

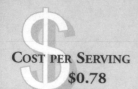

CHOCOLATE-BANANA SHAKE

PREPARATION TIME
5 minutes

SERVINGS 1

SERVING SIZE
1 cup

EXCHANGES/CHOICES
3 Carbohydrate

CALORIES 230
CALORIES FROM FAT 5

TOTAL FAT 1 g
SATURATED FAT <1 g
TRANS FAT 0 g

CHOLESTEROL 10 mg

SODIUM 210 mg

CARBOHYDRATE 28 g
DIETARY FIBER 11 g
SUGARS 18 g

PROTEIN 11 g

This frosty recipe for one can be doubled to serve a friend too!

1/4 cup fat-free milk
1 cup fat-free sugar-free vanilla ice cream
1 Tbsp sugar-free instant chocolate milk mix
1/4 medium ripe banana (a medium banana weighs
  approximately 6 oz with peel)

1. Place all ingredients in blender and blend until thick
   and smooth.

WILD BERRY SYRUP

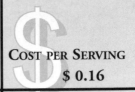
This syrup is delicious over Cinnamon French Toast,
p. 85, pancakes, waffles, or sugar-free ice cream.

1 cup water
1 0.3-oz package sugar-free wild berry-flavored–gelatin
1 12-oz package fresh blueberries or unsweetened frozen
   blueberries, thawed
1/2 cup cold water
1 1/2 Tbsp cornstarch

1. In a large saucepan, bring 1 cup water to a boil. Add
   gelatin and whisk until dissolved. Stir in blueberries,
   reduce heat to medium, bring to a simmer, and cook
   uncovered for 5 minutes.

2. In a liquid measuring cup, combine cold water and
   cornstarch, stirring until cornstarch is dissolved. Add
   cornstarch mixture to berry mixture, increase heat to
   high, bring to a boil, and cook 1 minute, whisking
   constantly.

3. Place 1 cup of mixture in blender, cover, and process
   until smooth. Pour fruit puree into a serving container,
   then stir in remaining blueberry mixture. Serve warm.
   Refrigerate leftovers—will gel with cooling.

PREPARATION TIME
10 minutes

COOKING TIME
15 minutes

SERVINGS 20

SERVING SIZE
2 Tbsp

EXCHANGES/CHOICES
1 Free food

CALORIES 15
CALORIES FROM FAT 0

TOTAL FAT 0 g
SATURATED FAT 0 g
TRANS FAT 0 g

CHOLESTEROL 0 mg

SODIUM 10 mg

CARBOHYDRATE 3 g
DIETARY FIBER 0 g
SUGARS 2 g

PROTEIN 0 g

INDEX

ALPHABETICAL LIST OF RECIPES

SUBJECT INDEX

A

Alcoholic beverages, 8, 54, 71
American Association of Diabetes
    Educators, 12
American Diabetes Association
    contact information, 12
    Diabetes Food Pyramid. *see*
        Diabetes Food Pyramid
    nutrition recommendations, 2, 9–11
American Dietetic Association
    average daily food cost, 3
    contact information, 12
Appetizers, 71

B

Bad buys, 40
Batch cooking, 22
Beans, 20, 46–47
Best buys, 40
    fruits, 50
    grains/beans/starchy vegetables, 46
    meat/protein, 52
    milk, 51
    vegetables, 46, 48
Beverages, 55
    alcoholic, 8, 54, 71
    eating out and, 69
Bread, 46–47
Buttermilk, 51

C

Calories, 9
Canned goods, 23, 49, 50
Carbohydrate counting, 17
Carbohydrates, 7–8, 10
Casseroles, 23
    quick six plan, 30–31
    safe handling of, 23, 24
Cereal, 46
Certified diabetes educators (CDEs), 12
Cheese, 52–53

Chicken, 52–53, 69
Cholesterol, 10
Container herb gardens, 62
Convenience foods, 41, 49
Cooking, cost-wise, 20, 22–23
    with fresh herbs, 61
Cooperative Extension Service offices,
    60, 62
Coupons, 38, 71

D

Dairy products, 7, 20, 51
DASH Eating Plan, 7
Defrosting foods, 23, 24
Deli meats, 40, 53
Diabetes, costs of, 1
Diabetes Control and Complications
    Trial (DCCT), 2
Diabetes Food Pyramid
    meal planning and, 17
    thrifty shopping tips, 45–57
        fats/sweets/alcohol, 54
        fruits, 50
        grains/beans/starchy
            vegetables, 46–47
        low-cost alternatives, 57
        meat and others, 52–53
        milk, 51
        miscellaneous foods, 55–56
        vegetables, 48–49
Diabetic foods, 2, 41, 54

E

Eating out, 67–72
    alcoholic beverages, 71
    appetizers, 71
    cost of, 67, 68
    coupon books, 71
    desserts, 71
    discount dining cards, 71
    downsizing, 72
    early-bird specials, 70
    ethnic restaurants, 70

Other Titles Available from the American Diabetes Association

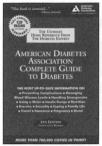

American Diabetes Association Complete Guide to Diabetes, 4th Edition
by American Diabetes Association
Have all the tips and information on diabetes that you need close at hand. The world's largest collection of diabetes self-care tips, techniques, and tricks for solving diabetes-related problems is back in its fourth edition, and it's bigger and better than ever before. **Order no. 4809-04; Price $29.95**

Holly Clegg's Trim & Terrific™ Diabetic Cooking
by Holly Clegg
Cookbook author Holly Clegg has teamed up with the American Diabetes Association to create a Trim & Terrific™ cookbook perfect for people with diabetes. With over 250 recipes, this collection is packed with meals that are quick, easy, and delicious. Forget the hassles of meal planning and rediscover the joys of great food! **Order no. 4883-01; Price $18.95**

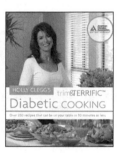

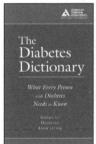

The Diabetes Dictionary
by American Diabetes Association
Diabetes can be a complicated disease; so to stay healthy, you need to understand the constantly growing vocabulary of diabetes research and treatment. The Diabetes Dictionary gives you the straight-forward definitions of diabetes terms and concepts that you need to successfully manage your disease. With more than 500 entries, this pocket-size book is an indispensable resource for every person with diabetes. **Order no. 5020-01; Price $5.95**

The 4-Ingredient Diabetes Cookbook
by Nancy S. Hughes
Making delicious meals doesn't have to be complicated, time-consuming, or expensive. You can create satisfying dishes using just four ingredients (or even fewer)! Make the most of your time and money. You'll be amazed at how much you can prepare with just a few simple ingredients. **Order no. 4662-01; Price $16.95**

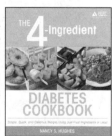

To order these and other great American Diabetes Association titles, call 1-800-232-6733 or visit *http://store.diabetes.org*. American Diabetes Association titles are also available in bookstore nationwide.

About the American Diabetes Association

The American Diabetes Association is the nation's leading voluntary health organization supporting diabetes research, information, and advocacy. Its mission is to prevent and cure diabetes and to improve the lives of all people affected by diabetes. The American Diabetes Association is the leading publisher of comprehensive diabetes information. Its huge library of practical and authoritative books for people with diabetes covers every aspect of self-care—cooking and nutrition, fitness, weight control, medications, complications, emotional issues, and general self-care.

To order American Diabetes Association books: Call 1-800-232-6733 or log on to *http://store.diabetes.org*

To join the American Diabetes Association: Call 1-800-806-7801 or log on to *www.diabetes.org/membership*

For more information about diabetes or ADA programs and services: Call 1-800-342-2383. E-mail: AskADA@diabetes.org or log on to *www.diabetes.org*

To locate an ADA/NCQA Recognized Provider of quality diabetes care in your area: *www.ncqa.org/dprp*

To find an ADA Recognized Education Program in your area: Call 1-800-342-2383. *www.diabetes.org/for-health-professionals-and-scientists/recognition/edrecognition.jsp*

To join the fight to increase funding for diabetes research, end discrimination, and improve insurance coverage: Call 1-800-342-2383. *www.diabetes.org/advocacy-and-legalresources/advocacy.jsp*

To find out how you can get involved with the programs in your community: Call 1-800-342-2383. See below for program Web addresses.

- *American Diabetes Month:* **educational activities aimed at those diagnosed with diabetes—month of November**. *www.diabetes.org/communityprograms-and-localevents/americandiabetesmonth.jsp*
- *American Diabetes Alert:* **annual public awareness campaign to find the undiagnosed—held the fourth Tuesday in March**. *www.diabetes.org/communityprograms-and-localevents/americandiabetesalert.jsp*
- *American Diabetes Association Latino Initiative:* **diabetes awareness program targeted to the Latino community.** *www.diabetes.org/communityprograms-and-localevents/latinos.jsp*
- *African American Program:* **diabetes awareness program targeted to the African American community**. *www.diabetes.org/communityprograms-and-localevents/africanamericans.jsp*
- *Awakening the Spirit:* **Pathways to Diabetes Prevention & Control: diabetes awareness program targeted to the Native American community**. *www.diabetes.org/communityprograms-and-localevents/nativeamericans.jsp*

To find out about an important research project regarding type 2 diabetes: *www.diabetes.org/diabetes-research/research-home.jsp*

To obtain information on making a planned gift or charitable bequest: Call 1-888-700-7029. *www.wpg.cc/stl/CDA/homepage/1,1006,509,00.html*

To make a donation or memorial contribution: Call 1-800-342-2383. *www.diabetes.org/support-the-cause/make-a-donation.jsp*